THE AETIOPATHOGENESIS
OF OSTEOARTHROSIS

THE AETIOPATHOGENESIS OF OSTEOARTHROSIS

Edited by

George Nuki
Professor of Rheumatology
University of Edinburgh

PITMAN MEDICAL

First published 1980

Catalogue Number 21–2624–81

Pitman Medical Publishing Co Ltd
PO Box 7, Tunbridge Wells,
Kent, TN1 1XH, England

Associated Companies

UNITED KINGDOM
Pitman Publishing Ltd, London
Focal Press Ltd, London

CANADA
Copp Clark Pitman, Toronto

USA
Fearon Pitman Publishers Inc, San Francisco
Focal Press Inc, New York

AUSTRALIA
Pitman Publishing Pty Ltd, Melbourne

NEW ZEALAND
Pitman Publishing NZ Ltd, Wellington

British Library Cataloguing in Publication Data

The aetiopathogenesis of osteoarthrosis.
  1. Osteoarthrosis
  I. Nuki, George
  616.7'2   RC933
ISBN 0–272–79434–1

Printed by offset-lithography and bound
in Great Britain at The Pitman Press, Bath

FOREWORD

For many years progress in understanding the aetiology and pathogenesis of osteoarthrosis was very slow. Research interest was severely limited by the concept that osteoarthrosis was a single disease resulting from attrition of articular cartilage by the inevitable processes of ageing, wear and tear.

This book presents a more hopeful and exciting prospect. Based on contributions to a small, multidisciplinary international symposium held at the Welsh National School of Medicine, evidence is presented that degenerative joint disease can result from the interaction of a wide variety of factors, some of which may eventually be subject to modulation.

The aetiopathogenesis of osteoarthrosis is examined by sophisticated modern morphological, biochemical and biomechanical experimental methods as well as by more traditional clinical and epidemiological approaches. The role of ageing and genetic factors are critically reviewed and recent work on biomechanical factors such as fatigue failure of the collagen fibre network and stiffening of subchondral bone as a result of microfractures induced by repetitive impulse loading are described. The sequence and consequences of biochemical and physicochemical changes in cartilage are considered as are cartilage changes induced by the synovium and its milieu. Evidence for an immunological basis for cartilage damage is presented and the possible roles of disordered mineral metabolism in cartilage, apatite extrusion and crystal synovitis are discussed.

The book would not have been possible without the financial support of the Arthritis and Rheumatism Council and May and Baker Ltd; the hard work of successive secretaries, Mrs Joanna Walker and Miss Dianne Clachan; the forebearance by colleagues and family and the persistent cheerful courtesy and efficiency of Mrs Betty Dickens of Pitman Medical.

George Nuki
Edinburgh 1979

LIST OF CONTRIBUTORS

S Y Ali   Experimental Pathology Unit, Institute of Orthopaedics, University of London, United Kingdom

C G Armstrong   Department of Mechanical Engineering, Queens University, Belfast, Northern Ireland

E L Bennett   Division of Orthopaedics, Queens University, Kingston, Ontario, Canada

T D V Cooke   Division of Orthopaedics, Queens University, Kingston, Ontario, Canada

P A Dieppe   St Bartholomew's Hospital, London, United Kingdom

M G Ehrlich   Department of Orthopaedics, Massachusetts General Hospital, Boston, USA

R J Elliott   Department of Histopathology, University of Manchester, United Kingdom

D Eyre   Orthopaedic Research Laboratory, Children's Hospital Medical Centre, Boston, Massachusetts, USA

H B Fell   Department of Pathology, University of Cambridge, United Kingdom

M A R Freeman   Department of Orthopaedic Surgery, The London Hospital, United Kingdom

D L Gardner   Department of Histopathology, University of Manchester, United Kingdom

P Harper   Department of Medicine, Welsh National School of Medicine, Cardiff, United Kingdom

D S Howell   Veterans Administration Hospital, University of Miami, Florida, USA

E C Huskisson   St Bartholomew's Hospital, London, United Kingdom

R W Jubb   Department of Pathology, University of Cambridge, United Kingdom

D A Kalbhen   Pharmakologisches Institut, University of Bonn, West Germany

J S Lawrence   Medizinisch Hochschule, Hannover, West Germany

R B Longmore   Department of Anatomy, University of Dundee, United Kingdom

G Lust — James A Baker Institute for Animal Health, Cornell University, Ithaca, New York, USA

C McDevitt — Division of Biochemistry, Kennedy Institute of Rheumatology, London, United Kingdom

H J Mankin — Department of Orthopaedics, Massachusetts General Hospital, Boston, USA

A Maroudas — Bone and Joint Research Unit, The London Hospital, United Kingdom

G Meachim — Department of Pathology, University of Liverpool, United Kingdom

D R Miller — James A Baker Institute for Animal Health, Cornell University, Ithaca, New York

H Muir — Division of Biochemistry, Kennedy Institute for Rheumatology, London, United Kingdom

G Nuki — Rheumatic Diseases Unit, University of Edinburgh, United Kingdom

O Ohno — Division of Orthopaedics, Queens University, Kingston, Ontario, Canada

I L Paul — Massachusetts Institute of Technology, Boston, USA

E L Radin — Department of Orthopaedic Surgery, West Virginia University Medical Center, Morgantown, USA

R M Rose — Massachusetts Institute of Technology, Boston, USA

M Sebo — Medizinisch Hochschule, Hannover, West Germany

L Sokoloff — State University of New York at Stony Brook, USA

M F Venn — Bone and Joint Research Unit, The London Hospital, United Kingdom

D A Willoughby — St Bartholomew's Hospital, London, United Kingdom

CONTENTS

1

THE PATHOLOGY OF OSTEOARTHROSIS AND THE ROLE OF AGEING

L Sokoloff

Osteoarthrosis is not a single disease. It results from a variety of patterns of joint failure. These can be summarised as deformations in which there is deterioration and mechanical loss of the articulating surface associated with a disturbance of the configuration of the joint related to a series of reparative phenomena which result in proliferation of new articular tissue at the margins and base of the joint (Figure 1). The sequence of these events and their mechanisms are not clearly established (Sokoloff, 1969). Although overly simplistic, it is useful to recognise two broad but distinct mechanisms that may be involved. One postulates that osteoarthrosis begins as an intrinsic senescent or other degeneration of articular cartilage; the other, that osteoarthrosis is caused by abnormal mechanical stresses acting on joints. In reality both are involved.

Pathological Anatomy

Roentgenographic studies of slab sections are a necessary part of pathological examination of osteoarthrotic joints as well as other skeletal specimens (Meachim, et al, 1972). For femoral heads, coronal slab sections approximately 0.8 cm thick are suitable (Figure 2). The osteoarthrotic lesions are so distorted that orientation may be difficult. A useful landmark in such cases is the calcar, the thick cortex on the posteromedial aspect of the femoral neck. The use of dilute Indian ink to stain minute breaks in the surface has been recommended to identify the earliest stages of fibrillation (Meachim, 1972).

Degeneration of the Cartilage Surface

The traditional description of the normal joint surface being very smooth has been re-examined by numerous investigators in recent years because of its importance in lubrication and wear in osteoarthrosis. It had been the belief that

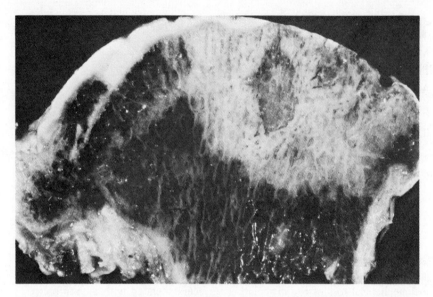

Figure 1   Advanced osteoarthrosis, head of femur. The contour is deformed both by loss
of white articular cartilage and by the formation of marginal osteophytes. The spur at
the left has grown not only to the side but superiorly onto the original joint surface. It
is capped by newly formed cartilage. Subchondral pseudocysts approach the joint
surface through slender crevices. The pallor of the eburnated tissue reflects the conden-
sation of bony trabeculae and fibrous tissue in contrast to the darker haematopoietic
marrow.

minute breaks in the surface, arising from collapse of lacunae of necrobiotic
('effete') chondrocytes were the site of the tears in fibrillation. Reflected light,
transmission and scanning electron microscopy, and tallysurf measurements
have been adduced to show that there normally is a degree of irregularity (Clarke,
1972; Gardner & Longmore, 1974; Meachim & Roy, 1969; Walker et al, 1968,
Zimny & Redler, 1974); that the irregularity increases with age and imperceptibly
goes over into fibrillation. There are significant technical limitations on the
validity of these measurements, mostly stemming from unavoidable dehydration
artifacts which result in collapse of the water-rich ground substance sols. The
data reported are often contradictory. The so-called lamina splendens, a putative
non collagenous layer forming the surface of the cartilage, may or may not be a
true structure. There are at present no techniques for distinguishing rigorously
between such a layer and an adsorbed film of synovial mucin. One recent scanning
electron microscopy study suggested that normal articular cartilage is relatively
smooth, but when the elastic properties of the deep portion of the cartilage are
reduced, the surface becomes unstable and rippled as the joint fluid flows over it
under load (Mow et al, 1974). The possibility that exaggeration of this process
might then be instrumental in initiating the fibrillation seems unlikely because
the postulated instabilities are by far too brief.

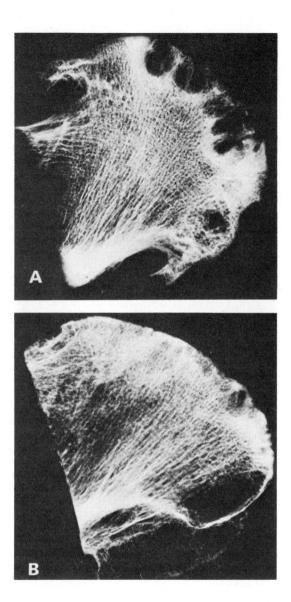

Figure 2   Roentgenograms of coronal slabs of femoral heads showing different config-
urations of osteoarthrotic deformity. The specimens are oriented as in situ. The superolateral surface is identified by the subjacent wedge-shaped spray of trabeculae. The
latter converge onto the thick inferomedial edge of the femoral neck. A – Numerous
subchondral pseudocysts are present, particularly on the superolateral aspect. The
osteophytes are small. B – Buttress osteophytes are present on both aspects of the
femoral neck. An enormous inferomedial osteophyte has merged with the adjacent
buttress so that the entire femoral head has assumed an externally ovoid configuration.
The surface is eburnated.

3

It has often been postulated that the superficial tangential layer is not only structurally different from the deepest layers of the cartilage (Weiss, 1973), but serves as an 'armour plate' in protecting the latter from mechanical injury (Mow et al, 1974). The only empirical data for testing this hypothesis, actual measurement of resistance to an artificial abrader in vitro, have given no support to it (Simon, 1971). Engineering analyses indicate that because friction is so low, articular cartilage is more likely to be damaged by impact than by abrasive forces (Radin et al, 1973). Detachment of articular cartilage first takes place at the tidemark, the interface between the non-calcified and calcified layers of the cartilage rather than at the osteoarticular junction (Hough et al, 1974).

There is one body of thought that suggests that the initial degenerative changes, or non-progressive ageing of joints, occur in relatively little stressed portions of the cartilage (Bullough et al, 1973). The bulk of the cartilage loss and exposure of underlying bone in osteoarthrosis ultimately is found in the more central rather than the peripheral portions of the joint surface. In the femoral head, it is most marked in the superolateral region. This corresponds to the wedge-shaped spray of trabeculae seen in roentgenograms (Figure 2) and usually is called the 'weight-bearing' portion. Weight is, of course, supported in different parts of the joint surface depending on the position of the extremity. It has been argued that the superolateral surface is not the point of maximal weight bearing; there are two singular points of maximum contact and initial fibrillation on the anterior and posterior surfaces, respectively instead (Bullough et al, 1973; Tillman, 1973).

The loss of joint surface is not confined to the cartilage. Subchondral bone also is eroded and polished. The latter, backed up by reactive new bone formation is responsible for the ivory-like (eburnated) appearance of the surface. Even in advanced eburnation, the exposed bony surface is perforated in many areas by nubbins of fibrous tissue and cartilage proliferating out of the subchondral marrow.

Necrosis of Bone in Osteoarthrosis

Two major patterns of bone necrosis are commonly seen in osteoarthrosis. One is a necrobiosis of osteocytes in the superficial layer of eburnated bone. It is conceivable that local frictional heat is responsible for killing the cells. The other is a more extensive segmental necrosis of subchondral bone. The latter most often results from minute fractures in the subchondral bone in areas of eburnation. These fractures are the rule rather than the exception in severe osteoarthrosis and probably account for much of the deformity even if they are not at the heart of the process (Storey, 1968; Storey & Landells, 1971). In other cases, focal areas of aseptic necrosis occur in which microfractures cannot be identified. Occlusion of minute intramedullary arteries has been demonstrated by angiography in such cases by Trueta. Nevertheless Streda's suggestion (Streda, 1971) that all osteoarthrosis of the hip is secondary to aseptic necrosis of the femoral head goes beyond the anatomical evidence.

Other events also shape the subchondral bone. The sequence usually taught, that bony changes are secondary to initial degeneration of the cartilage, may not be valid. A reshaping of the articular ends of the bones with age has been described repeatedly (Bullough et al, 1973). It has been proposed by some that this remodelling, when it exceeds the rate at which cartilage can accommodate to the change in shape, is the basic process in osteoarthrotic degeneration. Most of the published data on the subject have not come to grips with the problem of whether the surface of the cartilage has indeed remained intact while the bone changes its shape. Perhaps the best evidence for this comes from the temporomandibular joint, but the point remains moot. There can be no question that the changes in the osteochondral junction and reduplication of the tidemark do take place throughout adult life even in the absence of fibrillation (Green et al, 1970). The point is worth making because there is some engineering logic behind the thinking that articular cartilage is not a good shock absorber for impact loading, and that such impacts are the important events in causing osteoarthrosis (Radin et al, 1973). This places a greater importance on primary changes in the subchondral bone.

There is considerable variation in density of subchondral bone in osteoarthrosis. Aside from the eburnation and pseudocysts described below, there also are regions of osteoporosis. Daracott and Vernon-Roberts (1971) have emphasised the rarefaction of the subchondral plate as the anatomical feature distinguishing chondromalacia of the patella from ordinary osteoarthrotic fibrillation. In areas of remodelling bone in osteoarthrotic femoral heads, considerable osteoid material is found (Batra & Charnley, 1969). The new bone formation is the basis for increased uptake of bone-seeking isotopes in clinical scintigraphy of osteoarthrosis (Crutchlow, 1970).

Subchondral Pseuodcysts (Geodes)

Globoid or pyriform defects in subchondral bone are common in osteoarthrosis of the hip and the base of the thumb, but not in other joints (Gerber & Dixon, 1974).

The explanation offered for their occurence is that the joint surface supports extremely high pressures during weight-bearing, and that when localised discontinuities in the subchondral plate develop, pressure intrudes into the subchondral marrow and disturbs the circulation (Sokoloff, 1969). Three sorts of processes are seen histologically to account for the loss of bony tissue in the centre of these pseudocysts:

1. osteoclastic resorption associated with the formation of a fibromyxoid connective tissue (Figure 3);

2. localised osteoporosis, probably the least common form; and

3. necrosis and microfractures of the bone and adjacent marrow.

The centres of these areas contain fluid in only a relatively small percentage of

5

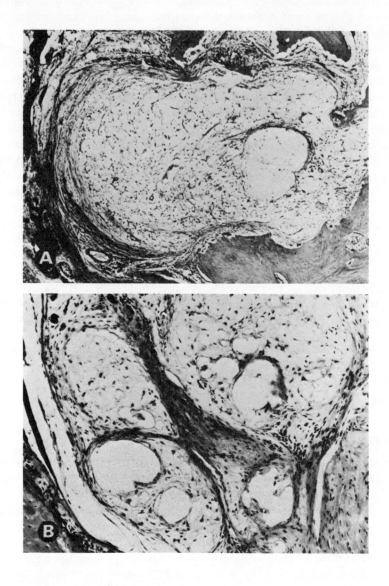

Figure 3   Mucoid pseudocysts in osteoarthrosis.
   A. Subchondral pseudocyst in human femoral head. A fibrous rim in forming at the periphery, and osteoclastic activity is seen in the adjacent bone. Haematoxylin and eosin stain.
   B. Early lesion in popliteal adipose tissue, 16-month-old STR/IN mouse. These mice have an inherited predisposition to severe degenerative joint disease. Haematoxylin and eosin stain.

cases. When present, the cysts form as puddles in the myxoid tissue and lack a synovial lining. They are morphologically similar to the periarticular cysts of Heberden's nodes and to ganglia. Rather similar pseudocysts are seen frequently about the knee of several laboratory rodents prone to osteoarthrosis. They form by liquefaction of the periarticular fibroadipose tissue rather than protrusion and pinching off of synovial pouches from the joint (Figure 3B).

The character of the cyst varies with the age of the lesion. Areas of haemorrhage are sometimes seen. The defect in the overlying bone plate is seen at the apex of the pseudocyst and often does not appear for this reason in random sections. The periphery of the geode is more cellular than the centre, and may be replaced by compact fibrous tissue, sometimes mixed with cartilage. External to these, congested sinusoidal vessels are common and new bone is laid down to form a sclerotic rim. The pseudocysts in the hip are larger on the acetabular than on the femoral side. They often are multiple and sometimes individually are more than 3 cm in diameter.

Structure of the Osteophyte

Osteophytes form in different locations of individual joints but share common pathogenetic sequences. Among the earliest seen are those growing into the marginal no-mans-land of cartilage, synovium, capsule, periosteum and subchondral bone plate. These often occur in regions where the immediately overlying cartilage is not eroded. At a later period, osteophytes may grow into ligamentous — capsular attachments to the joint, or protrude directly into the joint cavity. They are covered characteristically by a primarily fibrous cartilage and, peripherally by synovial fibrous tissue. The subchondral bone of the osteophyte is fragile. The surface of the osteophyte itself commonly is caught up in the osteoarthrotic process and becomes fibrillated and abraded. In the femoral heads, the osteophyte extends along the retinaculum and may merge with the cortex of the femoral neck (so-called buttress osteophyte Figure 2). At times the entire osteophyte and femoral head become so re-modelled that they form a single continuous ovoid structure. In the femoral head, osteophytes also form early about the fovea of the ligamentum teres but may become obliterated during progression of the eburnation.

Although the osteophyte may be regarded teleologically as an attempt to enlarge the bearing surface of the joint and thereby reduce pressure on it (pressure = force/area), it is also true that osteophytes interfere mechanically with excursions of the joint. Several prospective studies have demonstrated that small osteophytes often are present at the knee (Danielsson & Hernborg, 1970) and hip for long periods of time without apparent narrowing of the joint space or progressive deterioration. This is one of the reasons that have been offered for the belief held by some that ageing changes should be distinguished from osteoarthrosis. In evaluating this, it should be kept in mind that considerable anatomical destruction of joint cartilage may be present and not detected in conventional roentgenographic films. For this purpose it is desirable to examine the osteoarthrotic joint in a weight-bearing (erect) posture rather than while reclining.

Soft Tissues in Osteoarthrosis

Although degenerative joint disease by definition is not inherently inflammatory, focal areas of chronic synovitis and fibrosis are the rule in advanced cases. Mostly this is characterised by small focal infiltrates of lymphocytes and mononuclear cells in the retinaculum; occasionally it is sufficiently severe to raise a question of rheumatoid arthritis. A foreign body giant cell reaction to joint detritus also occurs and must be responsible for pain and effusion in acute cases. Secondary synovial osteochondromatosis is usually of minor degree. Synovial hypertrophy and fibrosis are the rule rather than the exception, and the synovium may appear quite villous in surgical material. Fibrous contracture of the capsule and ligaments contributes to the loss of mobility of the hip, and this forms the basis for older surgical procedures in which the ligaments were simply cut across. Amyloid deposits have been described in the capsule by one group of observers (Sorenson & Christensen, 1973). The ligamentum teres usually has disintegrated and is absent in resected specimens. In the knee joint, cruciate ligaments and menisci also become frayed, and a degree of instability results.

Heberden's nodes sometimes present primarily as para-articular mucoid cysts of the sort described above and come to the attention of the dermatologist. Recent experience has confirmed that these consistently arise in association with osteoarthrosis of the fingers; and that simple surgical excision of the cysts without removing at the same time the associated marginal osteophytes will result in recurrence of the cysts (Constant et al, 1969; Eaton et al, 1973; Kleinert et al, 1972). The cysts characteristically lack a synovial lining even though they may have communicated at one time with a joint.

Ageing

There are important semantic problems which must be grasped at the outset when considering ageing if one is to avoid ending in contradictions which are contradictions in philosophy rather than in substance. A recent workshop among experienced orthopaedic pathologists and systems analysts failed to devise a language for degenerative joint disease that would reconcile widely divergent concepts (Byers, 1975). Some used the term ageing of joints to indicate self-limited mild fibrillary changes or marginal osteophyte formation, while the term osteoarthrosis was restricted to the severely deformed, symptom-producing lesions (Byers et al, 1970). It may be more useful to regard senescence as the events in the articular cartilage that are associated with chrononological age exclusive of, and distinct from, osteoarthrosis itself. Ageing, however, is a loaded

8

word. Perhaps it is useful to consider two concepts; one of pathological ageing and one of biological ageing. Pathological ageing of joints can be further divided into what Byers calls progressive and non-progressive ageing changes. Thus overall there are three types of ageing phenomena in joints. Firstly there are age dependent histopathological changes which occur in all joints throughout the body. Secondly there are the progressive and destructive changes of osteoarthrosis which are part age dependent. Thirdly, there are time dependent changes in cells or matrix which are independent of fibrillation or osteoarthrosis which may or may not predispose to injury by mechanical trauma.

This third view of ageing provided the nucleus for the concept of 'degenerative joint disease' originally formulated by Walter Bauer and his colleagues (Bennett et al, 1942). Degenerative joint disease was seen to result from an increased susceptibility of articular cartilage to 'wear and tear' as a result of senescent deterioration not limited to articular cartilaginous tissues, occurring for example also in costal cartilage.

Cellular Senescence

It has long been taught that articular chondrocytes, following cessation of skeletal growth, are incapable of mitotic division. The assumption that these cells are unable to replicate themselves has been one of the premises on which the 'wear and tear' concept of osteoarthrosis has been based. According to this view, articular cartilage degenerates with age because the cells cannot replenish structural components which are depleted by mechanical strains. That this is not strictly true is suggested by the fact that clusters of chondrocytes are seen regularly at the margins of the fibrillated fronds and, to a lesser extent, deeper in the cartilage. The clusters have the appearance of newly proliferated clones, an interpretation supported by autoradiographic demonstration of thymidine incorporation by the cells (Hulth et al, 1962; Rothwell & Bentley, 1973). Furthermore, radiosulphate is taken up by these cells and deposited into matrix proteoglycans (Meachim & Collins, 1962).

An additional argument in favour of a replicative capability of chondrocytes is the formation of thick layers of cartilage about joint mice detached in cases of osteochondritis dissecans. Similar structures are seen at times in osteoarthrosis (Figure 4). This evidence is not too secure, because the possibility that the detached nidus was at one time displaced into synovial tissue and so evoked a cartilaginous proliferation cannot be excluded.

The ultimate proof that articular chondrocytes can indeed divide has come from in vitro cell culture studies. These are accomplished by freeing the cells through mechanical and enzymatic disintegration of the tissue, phenomena structurally analogous to the finding of chondrocyte clusters close to the edges of matrix-depleted or fibrillated cartilage in osteoarthrosis. The findings suggest that the failure of articular chondrocytes to divide in mature articular cartilage,

9

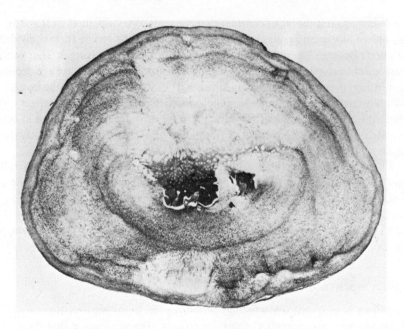

Figure 4   Proliferation of articular chondrocytes as shown in joint mouse from osteoarthrosis of the hip. Concentric layers of cartilage extend from the original joint surface
in the central nidus. Masson stain.

ordinarily, is not an inherent deficiency in the cells' replicating mechanism but results from their sequestration in a matrix that denies them access of macro-molecular growth factors. Dissolution of the matrix seems to be the stimulus required for the cells to divide. Articular chondrocytes have been grown with varying degrees of success from several mammalian species (Webber et al, 1977). Although in our hands human chondrocytes have failed to thrive under these conditions, there is no reason to believe that human osteoarthrosis results from a species — specific failure of its chondrocytes to behave like other animal types. Depending on the conditions of culture, rabbit chondrocytes faithfully recapitu-late in vitro both the proteoglycan profile (Srivastava et al, 1974) and collagen species (Norby et al, 1977) that are produced in vivo. Furthermore, cells from three-year-old rabbits divide and synthesise as much sulphated macromolecular material as do cells from young growing animals.

Articular chondrocytes contain proteases that can dissolve proteoglycans at neutral, naturally occurring pH (Sapolsky et al, 1964) as well as cathepsins and other hydrolases (Shoji & Granda, 1974) that have optimal activity at lower pH. The levels of catheptic activity are increased in osteoarthrotic lesions.

Matrix Changes

Articular cartilage, unlike most other tissues, is avascular and its cells are entirely dependent on a copious water-rich matrix for their metabolic exchanges. This necessitates a low turnover of cells and is nature's way of maintaining a structural stability of the bearing surface of the joints. The matrix is a composite material in which the fibrous component is collagen and the filler, the proteoglycan ground substance. The collagen is the source of the tissue's tensile strength; under conditions of health it turns over very little, if at all. By contrast, the ground substance is quite labile. The half life of chondroitin sulphate in rabbit cartilage is estimated as eight to 40 days; in man, 250 or more days (Maroudas, 1974). Because collagen persists throughout life, it is subject to slow molecular changes that may over the long run profoundly alter the physical properties of the tissue. There is an enormous literature on thermo-oxidation and cross-linking as mechanisms in the ageing of connective tissues (Herbage et al, 1972).

In osteoarthrotic fibrillation, the surface of the cartilage is disrupted, and there must necessarily be a disintegration of the pre-existing collagen fibrils in the tangential layer. As the lesions become more advanced, tearing of the collagen extends more deeply into the radial zone until ultimately the cartilage is sheared off. Microscopically the fibrils in the vicinity of the tears appear discontinuous, dishevelled, and unduly prominent ('unmasked'); these changes correspond to a diminution of the ground substance, which is readily confirmed histochemically and chemically (McDevitt, 1973). It is not possible morphologically to distinguish which of these intimately associated events, fatigue and disruption of the fibres or depletion of the proteoglycans, comes first. Experimentally these components may be modified individually by physical and chemical means, but one is soon followed by the other (Weightman et al, 1973).

'Unmasking' of the cartilage of older femoral head cartilage in the absence of overt fibrillation has been cited as an example of age changes in cartilage (Vignon et al, 1974). Unmasking and straightening of fibrils has often been referred to as amianthoid or asbestoid degeneration in this tissue by analogy to the fibrillary degeneration seen in rib and laryngeal cartilages. The argyrophilia and enormous diameter of the collagen fibrils of true amianthoid degeneration (Hough et al, 1973) are, in our experience, not characteristic of ageing or osteoarthrotic cartilage and have not been described in other accounts of the fine structure of this tissue (Weiss, 1973). The analysis of this phenomenon is complicated by the fact that reparative phenomena in osteoarthrotic joints result in a largely fibrous rather than a hyaline cartilage. Thus reports of a Type I molecular species of collagen in osteoarthrotic cartilage are difficult to interpret because the latter was obtained from surgically excised femoral heads (Nimni & Deshmukh, 1973). Lesions so severe as to require joint replacement lack the original joint surface, and cartilage available for study in them must be obtained from the osteophyte. This phenomenon must also be reckoned with in many other chemical analyses of osteoarthrotic tissues. This sort of sampling problem probably accounts for major disparities between the findings on proteoglycan synthesis and composition reported in this disorder (Hjertquist & Lempberg, 1972).

11

For operational purposes fibrillation may be considered the starting point of osteoarthrosis. Most chemical (Hjertquist & Lempberg, 1972; Maroudas et al, 1973), physical (Kempson et al, 1970, 1971) and morphological (Sokoloff, 1969) findings are associated more with fibrillation than with age changes in intact portions of the joint cartilage. Nevertheless, even if in general one cannot identify age-dependent changes in the absence of fibrillation, the concept of cartilage senescence distinct from osteoarthrosis provides a worthwhile handle for investigating the problem of biological ageing. One age-dependent change of this sort has been found: senescent pigmentation of the cartilage (Van der Korst et al, 1968). A golden brown pigment which is visible in cross sections but not in longitudinal sections of tendons, because of the optical orientation of the collagen, is detected in a much lesser degree in articular cartilage. Recent studies designed to elucidate the nature of this senescent pigment (Van der Korst et al, 1977) suggest that it is not lipofusein of the sort seen in epithelial tissues as a function of ageing. Pigmentation of articular cartilage progresses at a different rate from that observed in tendon and costal cartilage, reflecting the fact that articular cartilage is biologically very different from the other connective tissues. Its unique position in apposition with a joint space allows diffusion and turnover of small molecules not possible in other connective tissues. Clearly one cannot study the process of ageing in costal cartilage or tendon and simply extrapolate the results to articular cartilage.

To what extent is the distinction between progressive osteoarthrosis and non-progressive ageing changes in articular cartilage a real one? The thrust of the papers by Bennett and Bauer (1942) was that osteoarthrosis was simply the ultimate extension of a linear progression of ageing changes in joints. In an attempt to examine this question in a quasi quantitative fashion I have examined the nature of the ageing curve for human patella and femoral head cartilage using some maps of degenerative changes in the patella kindly supplied by George Meachim and some unpublished data from hips. Degeneration scores were constructed which placed equal weight on the amount of fibrillation, the amount of erosional wear and the extent of osteophyte formation by measuring the percentage of the surface that was fibrillated, the percentage of the surface that was eroded to the bone and twice the area of the osteophytes relative to the total surface. When the data for femoral head and patella were compared with autopsy data from the general population it was found that there was indeed a linear progression of degeneration after the first decade of life. This progression was more severe in the patello-femoral joint of the knee than in the hip. Linear progression of degenerative changes in the patella with age lead to histopathological changes that would be generally accepted as incontrovertable evidence of osteoarthrosis within a normal lifespan. On the other hand the rate of linear progression of degeneration in the femoral head in the general population was such that the curve would have to be extrapolated to about 200 years before the ageing changes progressed to what would constitute clinical osteoarthrosis.

Clearly there must be local factors in addition to simple pathological ageing involved in the pathogenesis of osteoarthrosis of the hip.

Repair of Osteoarthrosis

A limited potential for replication of chondrocytes in adult articular cartilage has already been noted, and so has the fact that new cartilage commonly is formed as part of the callus reaction in the subchondral marrow (Meachim & Osborne, 1970). The question has therefore been asked with increasing frequency whether repair or renewal in osteoarthrosis is possible. Numerous examples of an increase in roentgenological joint space, suggesting formation of a new cartilage, have been reported clinically (Perry et al, 1972). All recent experimental information (Campbell, 1969; Riddle, 1970) is in agreement with older findings that surface wounds in articular cartilage do not fill in, but that defects extending into subchondral bone repair to varying degrees of perfection. Surprisingly little anatomical material from human subjects following osteotomies or shaving of articular cartilage (as is sometimes done for chondromalacia patellae) has been reported. What there is indicates only at best a fibrous and new fibrocartilaginous repair (Byers, 1974). It is likely that much of the apparent increase in the joint space in roentgenographic films is the result of the angle of exposure rather than a measure of the cartilage regenerated. Subchondral pseudocysts and osteophytes, once formed, persist indefinitely.

It would be an error to conclude from these facts that there is no inherent potential for joints to repair themselves. Many clinical attempts are being made to influence the course of osteoarthrosis by stimulating the chondrocytes to synthesise ground substance or to retard its degradation by medical means (Chrisman et al, 1972). A priori there is no reason for believing that administering surrogate ground substance materials intra articularly or systemically, or even stimulating the production of natural ground substance in itself, would offer an advantage to the osteoarthrotic patient. The key to the repair of cartilage would seem to be that the chondrocytes can fulfil themselves only when there is a proper coupling of removal with synthesis of matrix, and necessarily too under conditions where the cartilage is not being subjected to mechanical insults as it is being formed.

In conclusion one must re-emphasise that osteoarthrosis is not a single disease but a pattern of biomechanical failure of joints. One or more components of the interacting mechanical and biological feedback loops may lead to a malfunction of this complex system. Biological modifiers have variable net effects depending on the particular target and timing of their actions.

Acknowledgements

Figure 1 reproduced with permission from Sokoloff, L (1972). The pathology and pathogenesis of osteoarthritis. In Arthritis and Allied Conditions. Eds. JL Hollander and DJ McCarty, Jr. 8th Ed. Lea and Febiger, Philadelphia.

Figures 2, 3, 4 and a large part of the text reproduced with permission from Sokoloff, L (1976) Osteoarthritis. In Bones and Joints: International Academy of Pathology Monograph N. 17 Chapter 8. Williams and Wilkins, Baltimore.

References

Batra, HC and Charnley, J (1969). *Journal of Bone and Joint Surgery, 51B,* 366

Bennett, GA, Waine, H, and Bauer, W (1942). *Changes in the knee joint at various ages: with particular reference to the nature and development of degenerative joint disease.* Commonwealth Fund. New York.

Bullough, P, Goodfellow, J and O'Connor, J (1973). *Journal of Bone and Joint Surgery, 55B,* 746

Byers, PD (1975).*Annals of the Rheumatic Diseases, 34,* Suppl. 147

Byers, PD (1974).*Journal of Bone and Joint Surgery, 56B,* 279

Byers, PD, Contepomi, CA and Farkas, TA (1972). *Annals of the Rheumatic Diseases, 29,* 15

Campbell, CJ (1969). *Clinical Orthopaedics, 64,* 45

Chrisman, OD, Snook, GA and Wilson, TC (1972). *Clinical Orthopaedics, 84,* 193

Clarke, IC (1972). *Annals of Biomedical Engineering, 1,* 31

Constant, E, Royer, JR, Pollard, RJ, Larsen, RD and Posch, JL (1969). *Plastic and Reconstructive Surgery, 43,* 241

Crutchlow, WP (1970). *Roentgenology, Radium Therapy and Nuclear Medicine, 109,* 803

Danielsson, L, and Hernborg, J (1970). *Clinical Orthopaedics, 69,* 302

Darracott, J and Vernon-Roberts, B (1971). *Rheumatology and Physical Medicine, 11,* 175

Eaton, RG, Dobranski, AI and Littler, JW (1973). *Journal of Bone and Joint Surgery, 55A,* 570

Gardner, DL and Longmore, RB (1974). In *Normal and Osteoarthrotic Articular Cartilage.* (Ed) SY Ali, MW Elves and DH Leaback. Institute of Orthopaedics, London. Page 141

Gerber, NJ and Dixon, A St.J (1974). *Arthritis and Rheumatism, 3,* 323

Green, WT Jr., Martin, GN, Eanes, ED and Sokoloff, L (1970). *Archives of Pathology, 90,* 151

Herbage, D, Huc, A, Chabrand, D and Chapuy, MC (1972).*Biochimica Biophysica Acta, 271,* 339

Hjertquist, SO and Lempberg, R (1972). *Calcified Tissue Research, 10,* 223

Hough, AJ, Banfield, WG, Mottram, FC and Sokoloff, L (1974). *Laboratory Investigation, 31,* 685

Hough, AJ, Mottram, FC and Sokoloff, L (1973). *American Journal of Pathology, 73,* 201

Hulth, A, Lindberg, L and Telhag, H (1972). *Clinical Orthopaedics, 84,* 197

Kempson, GE, Muir, H, Swanson, SAV and Freeman, MAR (1970). *Biochemistry Biophysics Acta, 215,* 70

Kempson, GE, Muir, H, Swanson, SAV and Freeman, MAR (1970).*Biochimica Biophysica Acta, 215,* 70

Kleinert, HE, Kutz, JE, Fishman, JH and McCraw, LH (1972). *Journal of Bone and Joint Surgery, 54A,* 1455

Maroudas, A (1974). In *Normal and Osteoarthrotic Cartilage.* (Ed) SY Ali, MW Elves, DH Leaback. Institute of Orthopaedics, London. Page 33

Maroudas, A, Evans, H and Almeida, L (1973). *Annals of the Rheumatic Diseases, 32,* 1

McDevitt, CA (1973). *Annals of the Rheumatic Diseases, 32,* 364

Meachim, G (1972). *Annals of the Rheumatic Diseases, 31,* 457

Meachim, G and Collins, DH (1962). *Annals of the Rheumatic Diseases, 21,* 45

Meachim, G, Hardinge, K and Williams, DR (1972). *British Journal of Radiology, 45,* 670

Meachim, G and Osborne, GV (1970). *Journal of Pathology, 102,* 1

Meachim, G and Roy, S (1969). *Journal of Bone and Joint Surgery, 51B*, 529

Mow, VC, Lai, WM, Eisenfeld, J and Redler, I (1974). *Journal of Biomechanics, 7*, 457

Nimni, M and Deshmukh, K (1973). *Science, 181*, 751

Norby, DP, Malemud, CJ and Sokoloff, L (1977).*Arthritis and Rheumatism, 20*, 709

Perry, GH, Smith, MJG and Whiteside, CG (1972). *Annals of the Rheumatic Diseases, 31*, 440

Radin, EL, Parker, HG, Pugh, JW, Steinberg, RS, Paul, IL and Rose, RM (1973). *Journal of Biomechanics, 6*, 51

Riddle, WE, Jr. (1970). *Journal of the American Veterinary Medical Association, 157*, 1471

Rothwell, AG and Bentley, G (1973). *Journal of Bone and Joint Surgery, 55B*, 588

Sapolsky, AI, Howell, DS and Woessner, JF, Jr. (1974).*Journal of Clinical Investigation, 53*, 1044

Shoji, H and Granda, JL (1974). *Clinical Orthopaedics, 99*, 293

Simon, WH (1971). *Journal of Biomechanics, 4*, 379

Sokoloff, L (1969). *The Biology of Degenerative Joint Disease.* University of Chicago Press, Chicago

Sorenson, KH and Christensen, HE (1973). *Acta Orthopaedica Scandinavica, 44*, 460

Srivastava, VML, Malemud, CJ and Sokoloff, L (1974). *Connective Tissue Research, 2*, 127

Storey, GO (1968). *Proceedings of the Royal Society of Medicine, 61*, 961

Storey, GO and Landells, JW (1971). *Annals of the Rheumatic Diseases, 30*, 406

Streda, A (1971). *Acta Universitatis Carolinae (Medical Monograph) Prague*

Tillman, B (1973). *Zeitschrift für Orthopadie, 111*, 23

Van der Korst, JK, Sokoloff, L and Miller, EJ (1968). *Archives of Pathology, 86*, 40

Van der Korst, JK, Willekens, FLH, Lansink, GW and Henrichs, AMA (1977). *American Journal of Pathology, 89*, 605

Vignon, E, Arlot, M, Meunier, P and Vignon, G (1974). *Clinical Orthopaedics, 103*, 269

Walker, PS, Dowson, D, Longfield, MD and Wright, V (1968). *Annals of the Rheumatic Diseases, 27*, 512

Webber, RJ, Malemud, CJ and Sokoloff, L (1977). *Calcified Tissue Research, 23*, 61

Weightman, BO, Freeman, MAR and Swanson, SAV (1973). *Nature, 244*, 303

Weiss, C (1973). *Federation Proceedings, 32*, 1459

Zimny, ML and Redler, I (1974). *Zeitschrift fur Zellforschung und mikroskopische Anatomie, 147*, 163

2

WAYS OF CARTILAGE BREAKDOWN IN
HUMAN AND EXPERIMENTAL OSTEOARTHROSIS

G Meachim

The morphological changes have been analysed in a series of 450 surgical excision specimens, mainly femoral heads, submitted for routine laboratory examination accompanied by a clinical diagnosis of osteoarthrosis in patients from Liverpool and North Wales. This analysis confirms the dual, or even triple, nature of osteoarthrosis in man (Figure 1). There is a destructive element, evidenced by a site of cartilage breakdown leading to bone exposure and bone wear

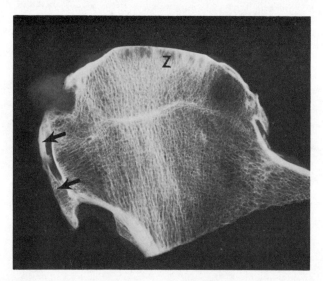

Figure 1. Osteoarthritic femoral head with cartilage loss and destructive flattening of the original bony contour on the zenith (z) contrasting with inferomedial remodelling by bony expansion (arrows). Osteophytic lipping is also seen, as outgrowths of new bone beyond the original perimeter of the cartilage. Note the subarticular osteosclerosis, interspersed with small osteolytic foci, on the zenith. Mid-coronal slab radiograph. This and all subsequent illustrations are of material from human joints

at this site. Elsewhere on the same specimen there is, in contrast, remodelling, with a variable amount of osteophytic para-articular lipping and of bony expansion of the original articular contour (Figure 1). In some specimens there is also a third, reparative element, seen as attempts to re-cover the exposed bone site by a surface layer of new non-osseous tissue.

The account which follows concerns only the destructive element in osteoarthrosis. In man this is characterised by progressive cartilage breakdown potentially to expose bone (Figure 2) at a site where the bone will then be subjected

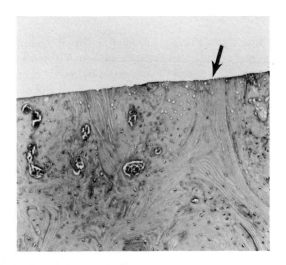

Figure 2. Characteristic histological appearance of osteoarthritic bone exposure in vertical section, with 'clean-cut' transection of a concentric lamellar system (arrow) and with empty osteocyte lacunae beneath the synovial interface. X 60

to abrasive and other damage. A progressive form of cartilage breakdown, leading to bone exposure, is also obtained in rabbit osteoarthrosis induced experimentally by intra-articular injection of papain (Bentley, 1971), and in naturally-occurring osteoarthrosis in hamsters (Meachim & Illman, 1967). In contrast, the lesions induced in rabbits by experimental scarification of cartilage (Meachim, 1963) lack a progressive potential towards bone exposure, and are thus not truly osteoarthritic in nature.

Late-stage Osteoarthrosis

In most surgical excision specimens from human osteoarthrosis, cartilage destruction has already progressed to the stage of bone exposure (Figure 2), or at least to exposure of the calcified cartilage layer (Figure 3), at the affected site. At this

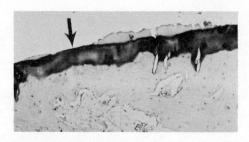

Figure 3. Severe destructive thinning of uncalcified cartilage (pale staining), with exposure (arrow) of the calcified layer (darker staining). Osteoarthritic femoral head. Toluidine blue X 60

site the exposed bone shows a typical histological pattern: its surface has a 'clean-cut' appearance, as if transected with a knife, and beneath the exposed surface there is a microscopic band of osteonecrosis, evidenced by a few rows of empty osteocyte lacunae (Figure 2); deep to this there is osseous remodelling activity in viable bone, predominantly osteosclerotic but often also with osteo-lytic foci. This histological appearance is characteristic of the destructive site in late-stage osteoarthrosis. It is seen both in primary osteoarthrosis, and in osteo-arthrosis secondary to causes such as rheumatoid disease. It occurs both in weight-bearing and in non-weight-bearing joints. The exposed bone surface is often interspersed with plugs of new fibrous or chondroid tissue.

At this late-stage of the disease, abrasive or grinding damage is an important factor in bone and cartilage destruction. Evidence for such damage is given by the 'clean-cut' appearance and trabecular transection (Figure 2) consistently seen on histology of the bone surface; by the macroscopic track markings seen on bone and cartilage surfaces from osteoarthritic joints in which movement was unidirectional, such markings being indicative of abrasive wear; and by certain features in shape and topography of vertical tissue slabs from osteo-arthritic joints (Meachim, 1972).

It should be emphasised that human surgical specimens from late-stage osteo-arthrosis do not give any direct information about the nature of osteoarthritic cartilage breakdown prior to the stage of calcified tissue exposure. This is because the cartilage from the crucial site which would give such information has by this stage developed full-thickness loss from the specimen: the evidence is no longer there to examine. Many workers have attempted to meet this problem by look-ing at the cartilage which still remains on the specimen, sampling, for example, the wedge-shaped cartilage segment (Figure 4) sometimes seen adjacent to the exposed bone area on a femoral head. However, it cannot be assumed that such cartilage necessarily recapitulates the morphological, biochemical and metabolic changes which occur prior to bone exposure. Instead, at least some of the changes in such samples could be the consequence of a local disturbance in their mechan-ical environment following the development of full-thickness cartilage loss else-where on the same articular surface.

18

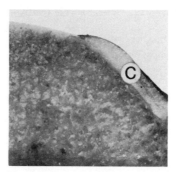

Figure 4. Part of a slab from an osteoarthritic femoral head, showing bone exposure (top left) with old cartilage (c) adjacent to this. Note the wedge shape of the cartilage at the junction with the exposed bone

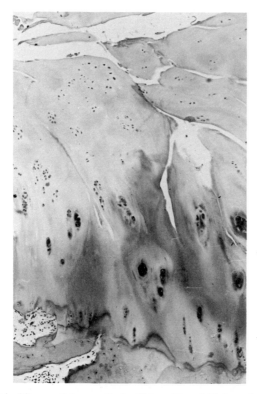

Figure 5. Tangential, oblique and deep vertical splitting of uncalcified cartilage, prior to bone exposure at the affected site. Zenith of osteoarthritic femoral head. Vertical section. X 60

19

Intermediate-stage Osteoarthritic Cartilage Breakdown

In a small minority of the series of surgical excision specimens of human osteo-arthritic femoral heads, cartilage destruction had not reached the stage of bone exposure. The difficulty in interpreting late-stage specimens could thus be partly overcome by examining this small group of intermediate-stage specimens, since they yield cartilage samples showing the lesions which occur in osteoarthritic cartilage breakdown on or near the femoral zenith prior to the stage of full-thickness cartilage loss at this crucial site. However, it should be made clear that no samples have been available from the acetabulum. The following types of intermediate-stage osteoarthritic cartilage breakdown have been observed:

1)   Disintegration and destructive thinning associated with deep splitting of *'fibrillation'* type (Figure 5). This sort of splitting follows the same alignments as those of cartilage collagen fibres, and, amongst other possible explanations,

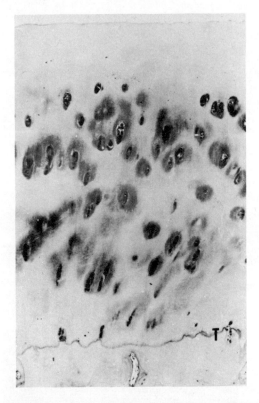

Figure 6. Thinned uncalcified cartilage with a virtually smooth synovial interface. Compare with Figure 5. Note also the cell necrosis (loss of nuclear staining) in the cartilage below the interface. Uncalcified-calcified junction (T). Zenith of osteoarthritic femoral head. Vertical section. X 60

would be consistent with a hypothetical 'fatigue failure' of the collagen frame-work (Freeman & Meachim, 1973). The concept of fatigue failure implies that a material has developed a mechanically-induced structural failure after repeated applications of loading of a magnitude which it was initially able to withstand without damage.

2)   Severe part-thickness loss of the uncalcified cartilage, but with no or only minor splitting apparent at the synovial interface of what remains of the matrix (Figure 6). This appearance of *smoother-surfaced destructive thinning* differs from that of typical fibrillation, and would instead be more consistent with 'abrasive wear' (i.e. 'grinding' damage during joint movement). It seems possible that this type of wear does not usually develop until after the affected cartilage segment has already been thinned by some other mechanism.

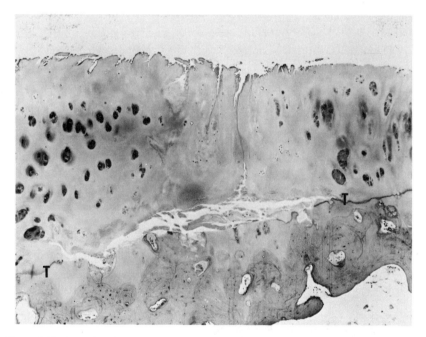

Figure 7. Horizontal cleft at the level of the junction (T) between uncalcified cartilage and its calcified layer. Note also the fine, vertical split from the synovial interface down to the horizontal cleft. Zenith of osteoarthritic femoral head. Vertical section. X 43

3)   *Horizontal splitting at the inerface between the uncalcified and calcified cartilage* (Figure 7). This would be consistent with 'shearing damage'. It perhaps results from excessive deformation (i.e. lateral flow) of the uncalcified matrix when moving under load, causing strainage of the anchoring between the deep uncalcified layer and the less deformable calcified layer. Following horizontal

splitting, there is evidence, from hamster osteoarthrosis (Meachim & Illman, 1967), that the overlying uncalcified segment can dissect away from its calcified base.

Deep splitting of fibrillation type, shearing damage, and abrasive wear are not mutually exclusive mechanisms of osteoarthritic cartilage breakdown, since each would tend to predispose to the other. In some specimens from intermediate stage osteoarthritis, two or more of the types of cartilage destruction described above have been noted on the same femoral zenith.

Although there is no important quantitative change in the collagen content of osteoarthritic cartilage, the histology of the intermediate-stage destructive lesions indicates, at least in the case of those of fibrillation type, a major structural damage to the fibre framework. There is also evidence of a reduced amount of proteoglycan and an increased water content in the matrix ground substance, and this proteoglycan depletion will increase the susceptibility of the fibre framework to further damage by mechanical effects. Several possible factors may contribute to the proteoglycan changes:

a)   Diminished synthesis of proteoglycans, due to chondrocyte necrosis;

b)   physical leakage from the matrix, due to inadequate enmeshment of proteoglycan molecules by the damaged collagen fibre framework;

c)   increased enzymatic degradation of proteoglycan, due to there being higher tissue levels of lysosomal enzymes of chondrocyte origin.

Evidence from experimental osteoarthritis in dogs (McDevitt & Muir, 1976) supports a suggestion that in human osteoarthrosis the chondrocytes alter their manufacture of proteoglycans to a sort more characteristic of immature than of normal adult cartilage.

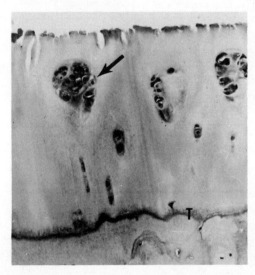

Figure 8
Thinned uncalcified cartilage with mainly shallow indentations at its synovial interface. Note the cell clusters (arrow). Uncalcified-calcified junction (T). Zenith of osteoarthritic femoral head. Vertical section.
X 150

22

Two contrasting changes can occur in the chondrocytes of cartilage segments undergoing osteoarthritic breakdown. There is cell necrosis (Figure 6), often widespread, but this change is sometimes accompanied by the formation of multicellular clusters by other, still viable cells (Figure 8). Such clusters are reactive in nature: they form by cell proliferation (Meachim & Collins, 1962) and are concerned in proteoglycan synthesis (Collins & McElligott, 1960) until they in turn eventually undergo necrosis. Reactive cluster formation can be induced experimentally in rabbits by cartilage scarification (Meachim, 1963).

Pre-clinical Osteoarthrosis

Although cartilage is now available for study from surgical specimens in the intermediate-stage of osteoarthrosis, surgical specimens are not, of course, obtainable for study of the nature of osteoarthritic breakdown of articular cartilage at the preclinical stage (Figure 9). The following comments can, however, be put forward as a basis for discussion of the preclinical lesions.

It is known that patients with osteoarthrosis are a heterogeneous group, and that osteoarthritic cartilage breakdown can follow a variety of predisposing causes.

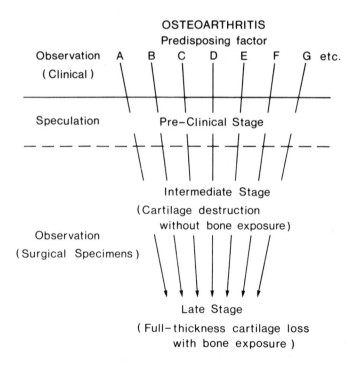

Figure 9. Diagram depicting clinical osteoarthritis as an end-product reached by a variety of pathogenic pathways from a variety of 'causes'

There is normally a relatively high resistance against the vertical progression of clinical breakdown towards bone exposure at a site where the bone will then be subjected to abrasive and other damage. Circumstances in which this resistance is overcome to give a clinical osteoarthrosis may be grouped under the following general headings, acting alone or in combination.

1)   Circumstances in which the cartilage has normal properties as a material but is subjected to an abnormal biomechanical environment due, for example, to an inherited or acquired anatomical abnormality such as congenital dislocation of the hip, or recurrent dislocation of the patella. These anatomical abnormalities perhaps act by causing dangerously high pressure contacts when the cartilage is under load.

This group of circumstances also includes changes in articular cartilage environment from bone infarction, from hypothetical disturbances in joint remodelling (Johnson, 1959), from hypothetical alterations in the resilience of the underlying bone and from hypothetical deficiency in the wear-protecting properties of synovial fluid.

2)   Circumstances in which the mechanical environment is initially normal, but the cartilage has an inherited or acquired deficiency in its wear resistance as a material. Examples here include osteoarthrosis following cartilage pigment accumulation in ochronosis, and following crystal deposition in pyrophosphate arthropathy. Osteoarthrosis superimposed on rheumatoid disease may also be assigned to this group, since in rheumatoid arthritis several changes impair the efficiency of cartilage as a protective covering material: 'erosive' loss of tissue by fibroblast or macrophage invasion of the cartilage; weakening of the collagen fibre framework due to proteoglycan depletion. However, in a late-stage rheumatoid joint an abnormal mechanical environment may be a further contributory element.

3)   Circumstances in which day-to-day wear of apparently normal cartilage has been sufficiently prolonged to give osteoarthritic bone exposure in older subjects. The age-related patello-femoral osteoarthrosis which commonly occurs in elderly Liverpool women would seem to be an example here.

Because of the heterogeneity of osteoarthrosis in man, it cannot be assumed that the nature of cartilage breakdown in the preclinical stage (Figure 9) is the same for each cause, nor assumed that osteoarthrosis of 'primary' type always follows the same pathogenic pathway from a single, predisposing (but as yet unknown) cause. In line with the heterogeneity of human osteoarthrosis, the disease can be induced experimentally in animals either by altering the mechanical environment of the cartilage, for example, following division of the cruciate ligament of the dog's knee (McDevitt & Muir, 1976), or by altering the wear resistance of the cartilage as material, for example, following intra-articular injection of papain in the rabbit (Bentley, 1971).

A multifactorial concept for the pathogenesis of cartilage breakdown in pre-

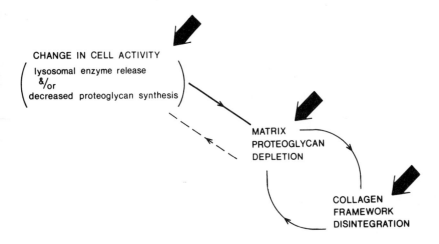

CHANGE IN CELL ACTIVITY

lysosomal enzyme release

&/or

decreased proteoglycan synthesis

MATRIX
PROTEOGLYCAN
DEPLETION

COLLAGEN
FRAMEWORK
DISINTEGRATION

Figure 10. The tendency for a vicious cycle in articular cartilage breakdown. Note that these are several possible initial modes of entry (broad arrows) into the cycle

clinical osteoarthrosis is supported by the concept of a functional interdependence in the constituents of cartilage as a tissue (Figure 10). 'Mechanical' and 'biochemical' hypotheses for the pathogenesis of osteoarthrosis are not mutually exclusive. The proteoglycans and the collagen of the extracellular matrix both make an important contribution to the mechanical properties of intact cartilage. Diminished synthesis or increased enzymatic degradation of proteoglycans, due to a change in cellular activity, will soften the matrix and thus indirectly weaken its fibre framework. Conversely, direct damage to the collagen framework will lead to changes in the ground substance. Moreover, collagen framework disintegration or ground substance proteoglycan depletion can adversely affect the environment of the cells, with a potential to alter or suppress chondrocyte activity. Thus a deterioration in any one of the interdependent components of cartilage will tend to set up a vicious cycle of cartilage breakdown, regardless of the initial mode of entry into the cycle (Figure 10). Therefore, the initial event in cartilage breakdown, whether naturally-occurring or experimentally induced, need not be the same in every case: deterioration in any one of the constituents of cartilage may each lead to further harmful changes in the material. Continued progression of such changes towards osteoarthritic bone exposure is, however, by no means inevitable. Thus whether or not the lesions remain bland or progress to clinically significant disease is probably determined partly by local factors in the cartilage segment concerned, such as the magnitude of compressive stresses in the case of weight-bearing joints, and partly by other unknown factors, as in the case of non-weight-bearing joints like those of the fingers in primary generalised osteoarthrosis.

Although the preclinical stage of human osteoarthritic cartilage breakdown cannot be studied by use of surgical excision specimens, cartilage samples showing mild degrees of deterioration are readily obtainable from adult joints at necropsy. Study of the natural history of these 'age-related' lesions suggests that many of them are not truly 'osteoarthritic' in nature, since many of them lack any major potential to progress towards bone exposure and clinically significant changes (Byers et al, 1970; Meachim, 1975). Even so, the morphology of certain of the cartilage lesions seen in human necropsy material is of interest, since some of the lesions may correspond to those which occur in the pre-clinical stage of truly osteoarthritic disease. In particular, studies using transmission electron microscopy (Meachim et al, 1974) have shown that one mild form of cartilage deterioration is characterised in man by ultrastructural separations within the collagen fibre framework of the superficial layer (Figures 11A and B), and there is evidence from other studies (Meachim, 1971) that a mild form of human cartilage damage can be associated with an increase in the thickness of the cartilage, consistent with collagen framework damage and an increase in water content. Here it is pertinent to note that there is evidence of cartilage collagen framework damage, together with biochemical changes in the pattern of matrix proteoglycan, at an early stage in the development of experimentally-induced osteoarthrosis in dogs (McDevitt & Muir, 1976). In man and in dogs, this matrix deterioration can be followed or accompanied by microscopic splitting and ridging at the articular surface (i.e. at the interface of cartilage and synovial fluid), giving the appearance termed 'minimal fibrillation' as seen on light microscopy.

Freeman and Meachim (1973) have suggested that one possible cause of age-related and of osteoarthritic breakdown of articular cartilage might be a hypothetical 'fatigue failure' of the collagen fibre framework. As already noted, the concept of fatigue failure implies that a material has developed a mechanically-induced structural failure after repeated applications of loading of a magnitude which it was initially able to withstand without damage. Such a failure might initially cause, in the pre-clinical stage, ultrastructural separations within the fibre framework (Figure 11A), perhaps accompanied by ultrastructural breaks in individual collagen fibres, and might then eventually lead to histologically apparent splitting and disintegration of the matrix of the sort seen in cartilage fibrillation.

Cartilage lesions in human necropsy material present a variety of appearances *en face* and in vertical section, strongly suggesting that more than one mechanism of damage is concerned in their pathogenesis. When examined from above by light microscopy, the surface markings of lesions of the sort termed 'minimal fibrillation' can show orientation of their *en face* directions (Meachim & Fergie, 1975). Orientation, when present, has been studied in relation to the *en face* alignment of the superficial layer of collagen. This study in man shows that orientation is often in a direction which, amongst other possible explanations, would be consistent with hypothetical fatigue failure of the collagen framework. Sometimes, however, the orientation is indicative of abrasive or adhesive wear,

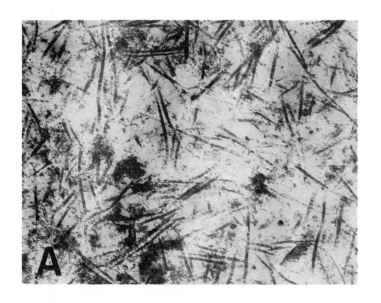

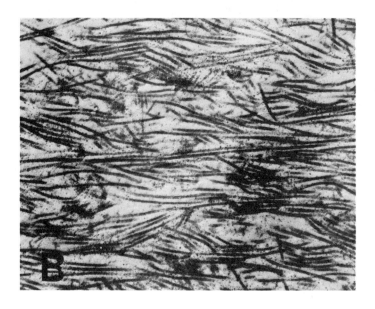

Figure 11. Transmission electron micrographs of sections cut tangential to the synovial interface, showing abnormally wide separation of the surface cartilage collagen fibres (A) compared with their appearance at an intact site (B) on the same articular surface. Necropsy specimen from the patellar groove of distal femur. X 25,000

with alignment in the direction of joint movement, and this second sort of wear can occur even in the absence of bone exposure on the opposing articular surface. 'Minimal fibrillation' is a clinically bland lesion which represents only a microscopic deterioration of the cartilage surface; however, it can in some instances lead to a further deterioration and thus to a histologically 'overt' fibrillation similar to that seen in surgical specimens from intermediate-stage osteoarthrosis.

'Minimal fibrillation' is seen histologically as a change at the articular surface. Recently, a further and different type of microscopic lesion has been studied in necropsy material: this is seen as tiny horizontal splits at the interface between the deep uncalcified and the calcified cartilage, and thus is a mild version of the calcified interface splitting sometimes observed (Figure 7) in surgical specimens from intermediate-stage osteoarthrosis.

References

Bentley, G (1971) *Journal of Bone and Joint Surgery, 53B,* 324
Byers, PD, Contepomi, CA and Farkas, TA (1970) *Annals of the Rheumatic Diseases, 29,* 15
Collins, DH and McElligott, TF (1960) *Annals of the Rheumatic Diseases, 19,* 318
Freeman, MAR and Meachim, G (1973) In *Adult Articular Cartilage.* (Ed) MAR Freeman. Pitman Medical, Tunbridge Wells. Page 287
Johnson, LC (1959) *Laboratory Investigation, 8,* 1233
McDevitt, CA and Muir, H (1976) *Journal of Bone and Joint Surgery, 58B,* 94
Meachim, G (1963) *Journal of Bone and Joint Surgery, 45B,* 150
Meachim, G (1971) *Annals of the Rheumatic Diseases, 30,* 43
Meachim, G (1972) *Journal of Pathology, 107,* 199
Meachim, G (1975) *Annals of the Rheumatic Diseases, 34, Suppt.2,* 122
Meachim, G and Collins, DH (1962) *Annals of the Rheumatic Diseases, 21,* 45
Meachim, G, Denham, D, Emery, IH and Wilkinson, PH (1974) *Journal of Anatomy, 118,* 101
Meachim, G and Fergie, IA (1975) *Journal of Pathology, 115,* 231
Meachim, G and Illman, O (1967) *Zeitschrift fur Versuchstierkunde, 9,* 33

3

BIOCHEMICAL CHANGES IN OSTEOARTHRITIS

Michael G Ehrlich and Henry J Mankin

The one agreed on feature of osteoarthritis is its inexorable nature. We all know that with time, the mildly symptomatic patient may progress to marked loss of motion and ultimately severe pain. Yet, clearly not all patients progress at the same rate, and there is some evidence that many do not progress at all. In reviewing the biochemical changes in osteoarthritis, I hope to indicate that the disease process represents an increasing conflict between repair and degradation, and that the ultimate fate of the disease represents the outcome of this conflict.

Proteoglycans

There is no question that there is a significant depletion of the proteoglycan content of the matrix. This has been established by the work of Bollet et al (1963), Anderson et al (1964) and Mankin and Lippiello (1970).

Confirmation of the quantitative data has also come from Maroudas et al (1973) who demonstrated a reduction in the fixed charge density. This reduction clearly implies a reduction in the proteoglycan content of the matrix since that macromolecule supplies most of the charge.

Since it was felt that the ionic charges bind the water (Linn & Sokoloff, 1965) this loss of proteoglycan content should have led to water loss, and therefore perhaps to loss of the resiliency or lubricating qualities of the cartilage, possibly permitting the remaining collagen fibres to be split (Radin et al, 1976) and to fissure. This splitting of the unprotected collagen fibres would, therefore, theoretically shear them off.

Actually, the problem is that several workers have found an increased amount of water content in cartilage above the 72–78% normally seen (Bollet, 1967; Mankin & Zarins, 1974). There is evidence both for and against this theory. Sokoloff (personal communication) has suggested that the clefts in the osteoarthritic cartilage may trap water which then fails to be removed by blotting and gives an artificially higher value.

Contrary to this, Mankin and Zarins (1974) have demonstrated that this increased water binding can be reduplicated by pre-treatment of the proteoglycan with 4M Guanidium hydrochloride. It is suggested that the removal of the proteoglycan permits binding to collagen fibres with greater affinity or allows the aggregates to expand and bind more water. They offered further proof for this by demonstrating that osteoarthritic cartilage had a greater binding affinity for water than normal.

If we have established that there is less proteoglycan, is this the result of diminished production? Actually starting with the work of Collins and McElligott (1960), and reinforced by that of Mankin and Lipiello (1970), Bollet (1967) and Mankin et al (1971), enhanced proteoglycan production has been repeatedly demonstrated. The increase in proteoglycan synthesis is up to twice that of normal cartilage, (Mankin and Lippiello, 1970) and this increase is proportional to the severity of the disease (Mankin et al, 1971) (Figure 1). Despite extensive data in this regard, this work has recently been challenged by Thompson (1977) who could not find a correlation with sulfate incorporation and grade of severity. The differences, however, may reflect the fact that Thompson used different sulfate washout techniques which could blur out differences.

It is highly significant that at a grade of 10, however, the repair process fails, and there is a sharp fall off in proteoglycan production.

Besides the total reduction in proteoglycan content, there is a question of change of type of glycosaminoglycan (GAG) or side chain produced. It has been suggested that the cartilage may revert to a chondroblastic stage, since work has

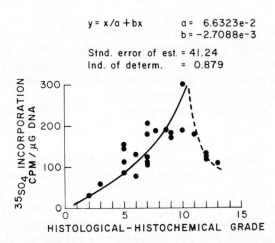

Figure 1   Radiosulfate incorporation in osteoarthritis. This progressively increases until a period of failure is reached. (From Mankin et al, 1971)

shown a relative decrease in keratan sulfate and increase in chondroitin 4:6 ratios (Mankin & Lippiello, 1971; Benmaman et al, 1969), both characteristic of the glycosaminoglycan production of immature cartilage (Mankin & Lippiello, 1971).

Hjertquist and Lempberg (1972) however, did not find this change in GAG composition. Bollet and his laboratory found shorter chain lengths suggesting hyaluronidase like enzymatic degradation (Bollet & Nance, 1966).

It is of interest that studies by Mankin's group (Mankin, 1975) do not show an increase in chondroitin-4-sulfate production in osteoarthritis, which might alternatively suggest that there is preferential degradation of keratan sulfate or chondroitin-6-sulfate.

Degradative Enzymes

If one then accepts the reduction in proteoglycan content, and the substantive data showing enhanced proteoglycan production, there must be enhanced degradation.

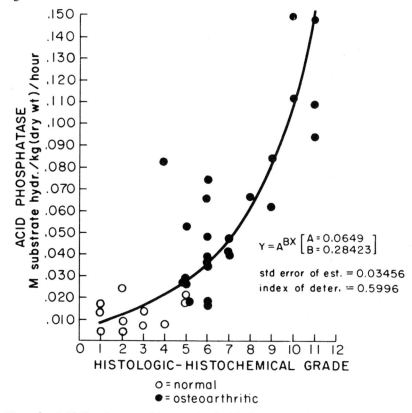

Figure 2   Acid Phosphatase activity correlated with the severity of the disease process. As the arthritis becomes more severe, the degradative enzyme level rises as well. (From Ehrlich et al, 1973)

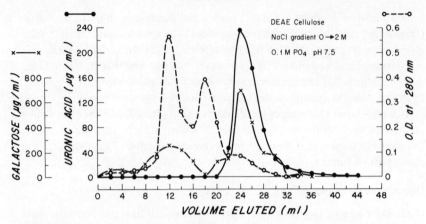

Figure 3   Breakdown products from proteoglycan subunit subjected to lysosomal enzymes at neutral pH. There are three large fragments. (Ehrlich et al, 1977a)

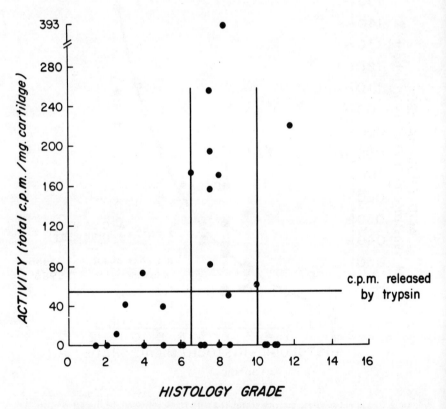

Figure 4   Collagenase activity in osteoarthritic femoral heads. There is very little activity with minimal or severe arthritis. (Ehrlich et al, 1977c)

Using acid phosphatase as a marker for lysosomal activity, and considering the focal nature of the disease, we studied 16μ sections of articular cartilage and found that in immediately adjacent sections, the enzymatic degradative activity was directly proportional to the degree of severity of the arthritis (Ehrlich et al, 1973) (Figure 2). This suggests that the cartilage contains the seeds of its own destruction.

Ali and Evans (1973) also demonstrated an increase in acid cathepsins in cartilage from osteoarthritic joints.

It has been demonstrated that acid cathepsins do have a hydrolytic effect on the protein part of the subunit (Sapolsky et al, 1973; Ali et al, 1967; Woessner, 1973). However, cathepsin D, the major protease affected, has minimal activity at pH7 (Barrett, 1975). Therefore, neutral proteoglycanase activity must be demonstrated. Woessner (1973) has demonstrated neutral proteoglycanase activity and we have shown that the lysosomal fraction of osteoarthritic human cartilage breaks down the proteoglycan as an endopeptidase releasing three large fragments (Ehrlich et al, 1977a) (Figure 3).

It is, therefore, suggested that with some insult to articular cartilage, a response is triggered which leads to the cartilage starting to degrade its own proteoglycan matrix, and at the same time trying to repair itself. Many factors could clearly tip this balance and ultimately lead to symptomatic disease.

Collagen

The other two components of articular cartilage are the collagen and the cells. It has been suggested that the collagen, might be mechanically degraded, since it is not present in end stage, osteoarthritis, and since several studies of osteoarthritis have shown that collagen content in unchanged (Anderson et al, 1964; Mankin & Lippiello, 1970).

However, recent work from our laboratory has demonstrated both that collagen production is increased in osteoarthritic articular cartilage (Lippiello et al, 1977) and that collagenase activity is present in the cartilage; the level of activity is proportionate to the severity of the disease to the point of failure (Ehrlich et al, 1977 b and 6) (Figure 4).

Chondrocyte proliferation

The final component to be considered is the cells themselves. As is well known, adult articular cartilage does not undergo mitotic activity (Mankin, 1963).

However, with osteoarthritis, there is a proliferation of cells, and in the early disease, the tissue is even hypercellular (Mankin & Lippiello, 1970; Hulth et al, 1972; Telhag, 1972). It is possible that the clones seen in osteoarthritis represent local areas of cell division. As with proteoglycan production, and collagen

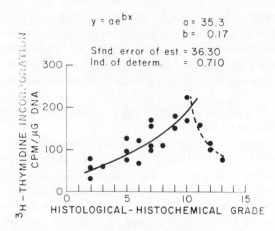

$$y = ae^{bx}$$

$a = 35.3$
$b = 0.17$

Stnd. error of est. = 36.30
Ind. of determ. = 0.710

Figure 5 ^{3}H-Thymidine incorporation in osteoarthritic cartilage. Cell division increases to a grade of 10, and then starts to decline. (From Mankin, et al, 1971)

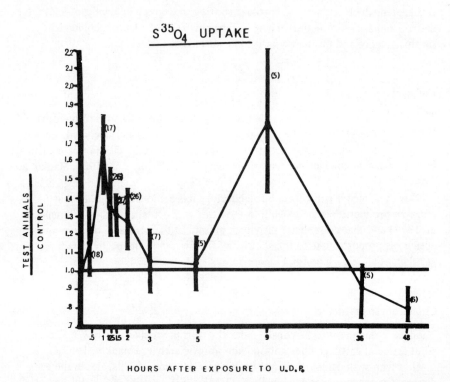

Figure 6 Uridine Diphosphate stimulation of radiosulfate uptake. There is a considerable stimulation of glycosaminoglycan production during the first two hours. (From Ehrlich et al, 1974)

production, the uptake of H-thymidine, a precursor of DNA synthesis, parallels increases in the severity of the arthritis to the point of failure (Mankin et al, 1971) (Figure 5).

Therefore, there is a balance between a constant state of reparative and degradative activity. To the point of failure, there are increases in proteoglycan, and collagen production and increased cell division. At the same time, both collagenase and lysosomal activity rises with increasing severity counteracting the reparative effects.

If there is to be a cure of osteoarthritis, it must come by something shifting the balance. This may come from altering the level of insult, e.g. osteotomy to change the surface bearing most of the weight, or from biochemical manipulation. For example, Sledge and McConaghey (1970) have shown that proteoglycan production can be stimulated by somatomedin and we have demonstrated that uridine diphosphate both in short and long term experiments can do the same thing (Ehrlich et al, 1974, 1975) (Figure 6). Perhaps a lysosomal stabiliser can accomplish the same thing.

Acknowledgments

Figures 1, 2, 5 and 6 are reproduced with permission of the publishers of the Journal of Bone and Joint Surgery.

The work was supported in part by a research grant (AM 16265–06) from the National Institute of Arthritis, Metabolism and Digestive Diseases.

References

Ali SY, Evans L and Stainthorpe E (1967) *Biochemical Journal, 105,* 549
Ali SY and Evans L (1973) *Federation Proceedings, 32,* 1494
Anderson CE, Ludowieg J, Harper H (1964) *Journal of Bone and Joint Surgery, 46A,* 1176
Barrett AJ (1975) In *Dynamics of Connective Tissue Macromolecules*
    Eds. PMC Burleigh, and AR Poole, North-Holland Publishing Co, Oxford. Page 200
Benmaman JD, Ludowieg JJ, Anderson CE (1969) *Clinical Biochemistry, 2,* 461
Bollet AJ, Handy JR, Sturgill BC (1963) *Journal of Clinical Investigation, 42,* 853
Bollet AJ and Nance JL (1966) *Journal of Clinical Investigation, 45,* 1170
Bollet AJ (1967) *Archives of Internal Medicine, 13,* 33
Collins DH, McElligott TF (1960) *Annals of the Rheumatic Diseases, 19,* 318
Ehrlich MG, Mankin HJ and Treadwell BV (1973) *Journal of Bone and Joint Surgery,*
    55A, 1068
Ehrlich MG, Mankin HJ, Treadwell BV and Jones H (1974) *Journal of Bone and Joint*
    Surgery, 56A, 1239
Ehrlich MG, Lippiello L, Mankin HJ, Higgins D and Knox O (1975) *Arthritis and*
    Rheumatism, 18, 396
Ehrlich MG, Mankin HJ, Vigliani G, Wright R and Crispen C (1977a) *Transactions of the*
    Orthopaedic Research Society, Las Vegas, Nevada
Ehrlich MG, Mankin HJ, Jones H, Wright R, Crispen C and Vigliani G (1977b) *Journal of*
    Clinical Investigation, 59, 226

Ehrlich MG, Vigliani G and Mankin HJ (1977c) *Transactions of the Orthopaedic Research Society,* Las Vegas, Nevada

Hjertquist SO and Lempberg R (1972) *Calcified Tissue Research, 10,* 223

Hulth A, Lindberg L and Telhag H (1972) *Clinical Orthopaedics, 84,* 197

Linn FC and Sokoloff L (1965) *Arthritis and Rheumatism, 8,* 481

Lippiello L, Hall D and Mankin HJ (1977) *Journal of Clinical Investigation, 59,* 593

Mankin HJ (1963) *Journal of Bone and Joint Surgery, 45A,* 529

Mankin HJ (1975) In *Dynamics of Connective Tissue Macromolecules.* Eds. PMC Burleigh, and AR Poole, North Holland Publishing Co, Oxford. Page 327

Mankin HJ, Dorfman H, Lippiello L (1971) *Journal of Bone and Joint Surgery, 53A,* 523

Mankin HJ, and Lippiello L (1970) *Journal of Bone and Joint Surgery, 52A,* 424

Mankin HJ and Lippiello L (1971) *Journal of Clinical Investigation, 50,* 1712

Mankin HJ and Zarins A (1974) *Transactions of the Orthopaedic Research Society,* Dallas, Texas

Maroudas A, Evans H, Almeida L (1973) *Annals of the Rheumatic Diseases, 32,* 1

Radin EL, Ehrlich MG, Weiss C, and Parker HG (1976) In *Recent Advances in Rheumatology, Part 1.* Eds. WW Buchanan and WC Dick, Churchill Livingstone, Edinburgh. Page 1

Sapolsky AI, Altman RD and Woessner JF (1973) *Journal of Clinical Investigation, 52,* 624

Sledge CB and McConaghey PD (1970) *Nature, 225,* 1249

Telhag H (1972) *Clinical Orthopaedics, 86,* 224

Thompson RC (1977) *Transactions of the Orthopaedic Research Society,* Las Vegas, Nevada

Woessner JF (1973) *Federation Proceedings, 32,* 1485

4

BIOCHEMICAL AND PHYSICO-CHEMICAL STUDIES ON OSTEOARTHROTIC CARTILAGE FROM THE HUMAN FEMORAL HEAD

A Maroudas and M F Venn

Introduction

It has often been said that it is not possible to study the progressive chemical changes in cartilage accompanying osteoarthrosis in man because one can only obtain joints in the advanced stages of the disease. However, if a sufficient number of femoral heads removed at operation for total hip replacement are examined, one does find that both the quantity of residual cartilage and its quality vary a great deal: at one end of the range there is little or no cartilage left; at the other end of the range one occasionally meets a specimen where the original cartilage is still present throughout the joint surface, covering even the superior region. In joints where a portion of the original tissue still remains, one observes considerable topographical variations in the properties of cartilage. These topographical variations may be related to the progress of degeneration. Thus it is likely that eroded cartilage adjacent to exposed bone represents a later stage of degeneration than does intact cartilage at a distance from the lesion.

With this in mind, the present authors have been examining the topographical variations in composition and metabolism of cartilage from osteoarthrotic femoral heads and comparing them with values for intact post-mortem material (Venn & Maroudas, 1977; Byers et al, 1977; Maroudas & Venn, 1977; Maroudas, 1976a). The present chapter reviews our various findings and conclusions, illustrating these with typical examples.

The effects of the changes in the composition of cartilage which occurs in osteoarthrosis on the physico-chemical properties are also discussed.

Results

Changes in the Chemical Composition of Cartilage in Osteoarthrosis

Hydration One of the most consistent observations on the biochemistry of osteo-arthrotic cartilage is that it has a higher water content than post-mortem cartilage (e.g. Bollet & Nance, 1966). An increase in hydration is also one of the earliest changes noted in experimental osteoarthrosis in the dog (McDevitt & Muir, 1976).

However, not only is the level of hydration increased in osteoarthrotic cartilage, but the pattern of variation with depth is often different from the normal with a maximum in the middle zone (Venn & Maroudas, 1977), as shown in Figure 1. Moreover osteoarthrotic cartilage usually swells when dissected from the joint and immersed in physiological saline whilst normal cartilage remains practically unaltered. The increase in the hydration of normal cartilage when excised from the joint and equilibrated in 0.15 M NaCl solution is around 1% and even in a hypotonic solution it does not swell by more than $1.5 - 3\%$. The degree of swelling is greatest in slices from the middle zone (Figure 2). It also increases if hypotonic saline is used as the equilibrant (Maroudas, 1976a; Maroudas & Venn, 1977).

The above phenomena can all be explained by a partial damage to the collagen network, which, as a result of this damage, is no longer able to restrain the swelling pressure of the proteoglycans (Maroudas, 1976a). In contrast to the osteoarthrotic specimens, the surface fibrillated cartilage from the perifoveal region of post-mortem femoral heads often shows an increased water content in the surface rather than in the middle zones (Venn, unpublished results); this would imply that in such cases collagen damage is more superficial, being limited to the regions closest to the articular surface.

On an osteoarthrotic femoral head one observes considerable topographical variations in the water content, related to the surface appearance of the tissue and the position relative to the lesion as shown in Table I (Byers et al, 1977).

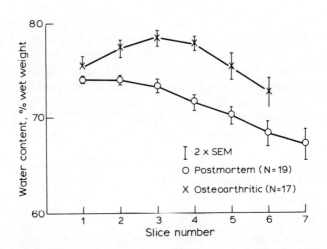

Figure 1 Typical Water Content profiles in normal and osteoarthrotic cartilage

38

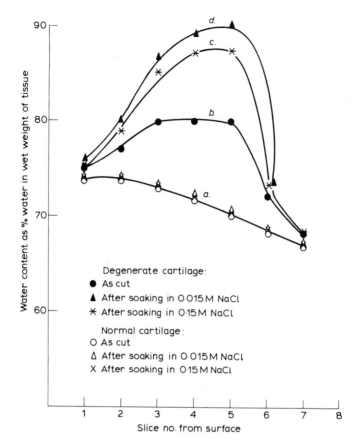

Figure 2 Variation in the swelling characteristics of normal and fibrillated cartilage with distance from articular surface (Maroudas, 1976a).

Visually intact cartilage, usually present at some distance from the lesion, has an only slightly raised water content compared with normal tissue. Cartilage showing coarse fibrillation, on the other hand, always exhibits a very high water content, though it is often present far from the areas of bone exposure.

The thin cartilage next to exposed bone has a higher water content than the corresponding zones of the visually intact cartilage.

Glycosaminoglycan content   Since the water content changes in degenerate cartilage, it is important to state clearly on what basis one chooses to express the chemical composition of the tissue. From the point of view of physicochemical and mechanical properties, it is the concentration of a given constituent either on a whole tissue basis or on a tissue water basis which is the relevant parameter. However, if one wishes to examine the changes in the absolute amounts of the

39

TABLE I Comparison between the composition and sulphate incorporation of normal and osteoarthrotic cartilage (Byers et al, 1977)

	Normal Femoral Heads		Osteoarthrotic Femoral Heads					
	Visually Intact Surface		Visually Intact Surface		Coarse Fibrillation		Fine Fibrillation (usually from zone of shelving cartilage)	
	Mean	SEM	Mean	SEM	Mean	SEM	Mean	SEM
Water content, % wet weight	70.9 ±	0.31	73.5 ±	0.66	79.6 ±	1.41	73.0 ±	0.5
Fixed charge density, meq/wet weight	0.153 ±	0.0038	0.129 ±	0.0061	0.068 ±	0.0065	0.094 ±	0.0067
Fixed charge density, meq/dry weight	5.26 ±	0.019	4.85 ±	0.045	3.33 ±	0.055	3.50 ±	0.041
Chondroitin sulphate, % wet weight	2.77 ±	0.06	2.36 ±	0.23	1.33 ±	0.16	1.54 ±	0.12
% dry weight	9.35 ±	0.33	8.90 ±	1.08	6.51 ±	1.23	5.70 ±	0.56
Keratan sulphate, % wet weight	2.14 ±	0.11	1.67 ±	0.18	0.88 ±	0.20	1.67 ±	0.22
% dry weight	7.35 ±	0.45	6.3 ±	0.82	4.30 ±	1.25	6.15 ±	0.92
Collagen content, % wet weight	17.40 ±	0.51	16.9 ±	2.49	14.85 ±	1.99	17.14 ±	1.44
% dry weight	60.0 ±	1.18	63.8 ±	7.82	72.8 ±	4.71	63.5 ±	3.4
Rate of sulphate incorporation, CPM/mgm wet tissue/5 hr	4,000 ±	600	3,500 ±	620	2,500 ±	700	2,900	
CPM/mgm dry tissue/5 hr	13,400	±2000	12,700	±2500	12,400	±4500	10,700	
CPM/mmole hexosamine/5 hr	40,000		43,000		56,000		44,000	
Calculated rate of synthesis of sulphated glycosaminoglycans, 106 x mmoles/hr/gm of wet tissue	0.5*		0.43		0.3		0.36	

* This corresponds to a mean turn-over time of three years for the sulphated glycosaminoglycans

various solid constituents as a result of degeneration, it is more appropriate to express results on a dry tissue basis. Table I gives the results of chemical analysis expressed in both ways. It should be noted that the values in this table are for unsliced chunks of tissue. Hence for cartilage excised from sites where the surface has been worn away a large fraction of the specimen will consist of deeper middle zone cartilage.

It can be seen that although in coarsely fibrillated cartilage there is significant loss of both chondroitin sulphate (CS) and keratan sulphate (KS) intact cartilage from an osteoarthrotic head shows almost the same CS level and only a slightly lower KS level than normal post-mortem tissue. Some visually intact specimens examined by us showed no divergence at all from the normal on a dry weight basis in either of these constituents (Maroudas & Venn, 1977; Venn, unpublished results) though there was usually a difference on a wet tissue basis because of increased hydration.

Specimens with a finely fibrillated surface showed an intermediate glycosamino-glycan content between those coarsely fibrillated and those with an intact surface whilst their water content was very close to that of the latter. It should be borne in mind, however, that cartilage with a finely fibrillated surface often came from thinned areas adjacent to exposed bone (Byers et al, 1977) so that comparison with full depth tissue from other areas is not strictly valid. Its low CS:KS ratio is characteristic of deep zone cartilage.

Sulphate Incorporation   As far as sulphate metabolism is concerned, the uptake, if expressed on a wet weight basis, is lower in all categories of cartilage from osteo-arthrotic heads as compared with intact cartilage from normal heads (Table I). If the results are expressed on a dry weight basis, however, there is no difference between the sulphate uptake of cartilage from osteoarthrotic femoral heads as compared with that from normal heads except in the zone of shelving cartilage where a considerable decrease is observed (Byers et al, 1977).

Effects of changes in chemical composition on physicochemical properties of cartilage

Because of the increased hydration almost invariably observed in osteoarthrotic cartilage, both the total glycosaminoglycan content and the fixed charge density when expressed on a total tissue basis are lower than in normal post-mortem cartilage (Table I) even before any actual loss has occurred. This leads to changes in several of the physicochemical properties of the tissue.

Hydraulic permeability   Recent measurements of the hydraulic permeability of visually intact cartilage from an osteoarthrotic femoral head show it to be some 50% higher than that of cartilage from a normal post-mortem femoral head. Typical results are shown in Table II.

TABLE II Comparison between the hydraulic permeability of typical visually intact specimens of cartilage obtained from (a) normal post-mortem femoral heads and (b) osteoarthrotic femoral heads

	Normal specimen (full-depth)	Osteoarthrotic specimen (full-depth)
% water content	70	75
Fixed charge density per gm of dry tissue (meq)	0.567	0.560
Fixed charge density per gm of wet tissue (meq)	0.170	0.140
Hydraulic permeability (cm^3 sec/gm)	1.6×10^{-13}	2.5×10^{-13}

Since the hydraulic permeability is very sensitive to the size of the 'pores' in the proteoglycan-water gel and hence to the glycosaminoglycan to water ratio (Maroudas, 1968; Maroudas, 1975a), it is not surprising to find it to be considerably higher in the more hydrated osteoarthrotic cartilage.

As the tissue becomes more fibrillated, with the resulting loss of proteoglycans, the hydraulic permeability is further increased.

Osmotic pressure   Both components of the osmotic pressure, viz. the ionic (Gibbs-Donnan) and the colloid (entropic), increase sharply with increased glycosaminoglycan concentration (Ogston, 1970; Maroudas, 1973; Maroudas, 1975a,b; Maroudas, 1976a). Accordingly, in osteoarthrotic cartilage one can anticipate a decrease in the total osmotic pressure as compared with normal. Preliminary results obtained using methods which have been described elsewhere (Maroudas, 1975b; Urban & Maroudas, 1977; Urban, 1977) confirm this conclusion. The ionic component of the osmotic pressure has been found to lie in the range 1 − 1.5 atmospheres in visually intact or very mildly fibrillated osteoarthrotic specimens as compared with 1.5 − 2 atmospheres in the case of cartilage from normal post-mortem femoral heads.

Solute transport   The transport of a given solute through cartilage is a function of the diffusion and the partition coefficients (Maroudas, 1968).

As far as small solutes are concerned (i.e. common nutrients), their diffusivities do not depend on the glycosaminoglycan content (Maroudas, 1968; Maroudas, 1975a). However, there is a slight effect of hydration; thus the diffusion coefficient of tritiated water is 10% higher in osteoarthrotic than in normal cartilage (Maroudas & Venn, 1977).

The partition coefficients of all solutes are directly proportional to the hydration of the tissue as this determines the available volume. However, as far as ionic solutes are concerned, a far more important factor is the fixed charge density (Maroudas, 1968; Maroudas, 1970; Maroudas, 1973). Thus, for instance, the permeability of osteoarthrotic cartilage to an electrolyte such as sodium sulphate is much higher than that of normal cartilage.

Large solutes such as serum albumin or IgG are practically excluded from normal femoral head cartilage (Maroudas, 1970; Maroudas, 1976b; Snowden & Maroudas, 1976). As the glycosaminoglycan concentration decreases, however, the permeability of cartilage to these solutes rapidly increases. Hence, as one would anticipate, some penetration of large solutes does occur into osteoarthrotic tissue (Maroudas, unpublished results).

General Discussion

Our work on human osteoarthrotic cartilage shows a great variation in the properties of the latter, depending on the surface characteristics of the tissue and its location on the joint. A considerable proportion of the cartilage examined shows properties very close to those observed in normal post-mortem cartilage. It thus appears that even in hips removed for total hip replacement there are specimens of cartilage at a very early stage of degeneration as well as at intermediate and late stages.

The finding that an increased water content is sometimes observed in specimens from osteoarthrotic heads which show no loss of glycosaminoglycans agrees with the results of McDevitt and Muir (1976) obtained in early stages of induced osteoarthritis in the dog.

Our view is that it is an impairment in the collagen network which leads to increased hydration, the network being no longer able to counteract the osmotic pressure of the proteoglycans as efficiently as in normal tissue (Maroudas et al, 1973; Maroudas, 1976a; Maroudas & Venn, 1977).

Our hypothesis is supported by the fact that whilst intact cartilage does not change its water content when the swelling pressure difference between it and the surrounding solution is altered, fibrillated tissue does swell when the osmotic stress is increased (Maroudas, 1976a). Thus, when a full depth chunk of surface fibrillated cartilage is excised from the joint and cut into thinner slices parallel to the articular surface, and these are allowed to equilibrate in buffered saline (0.15M NaCl), considerable swelling occurs in the slices from the middle zone, compared with the original water content. This is consistent with the increased osmotic stress in these slices when exposed directly to isotonic saline solution as compared with the situation in the uncut joint. Thus, it must be borne in mind that within the joint there is a gradual increase in the glycosaminoglycan content with distance from the articular surface and that it is the surface alone, with its low GAG concentration, which is in direct contact with synovial fluid. As a result, there is a gentle grading of osmotic stress within the tissue (Maroudas, 1976a). When cartilage is excised from the joint, however, and slices from each zone are exposed directly to saline solution, the swelling pressure gradient is considerably increased in regions where the glycosaminoglycan content is high. If the elastic restraining force of the collagen network is impaired in these regions, the increased osmotic pressure gradient leads to water imbibition.

A further proof that, once the collagen network is defective, it is the osmotic pressure gradient which determines the hydration level is provided by the fact that swelling is further increased when the same cartilage slices are re-equilibrated in a hypotonic solution. This leads to an increase in the ionic component of the pressure differential (e.g. Maroudas, 1975b).

It has been shown (Maroudas & Venn, 1977) that the increased water content in fibrillated cartilage is neither due to 'bound water' being present, as has been suggested in the literature (Mankin & Zarins-Thrasher, 1976), nor to disaggregated proteoglycans leading to increased osmotic pressure (Bollet & Nance, 1966).

It is still not known whether the primary event which leads to cartilage degeneration is glycosaminoglycan loss brought about enzymatically, with the damage to the collagen network following (Ali & Bayliss, 1974); or whether mechanical fatigue (Freeman & Meachim, 1973) is the direct cause of fibrillation, with the damaged collagen network subsequently enabling the proteoglycans to escape from the articular surface. The observation that in osteoarthrosis in the dog (McDevitt & Muir, 1976), and in some visually intact specimens of human osteoarthrotic cartilage removed for joint replacement, the water content is increased while the GAG levels often remain normal or nearly normal, suggests that collagen fatigue and breakdown may be the earliest in a destructive chain of events.

Whatever the nature of the first step, it is obvious that early swelling of cartilage must also lead, through dilution of GAG in the tissue, to increased hydraulic permeability and decreased osmotic pressure. This must create an unfavourable mechanical environment in subsequent stages of the self-destructive process outlined.

As far as changes in the chemical composition of osteoarthrotic cartilage are concerned, our results show a progressive loss of GAG, in agreement with the findings of other workers (e.g. Mathews, 1953; Bollet et al, 1963; Bollet & Nance, 1966; Mankin & Lippiello, 1971; Maroudas et al, 1973). There is some disagreement in the literature as to whether more KS than CS is lost or vice versa. Our results show a greater loss of KS, which agrees with the findings of Meachim and Stockwell (1973), Ali and Bayliss (1974) and McDevitt and Muir (1976).

The rate of glycosaminoglycan turn-over is of great relevance to the question of cartilage degradation and repair.

It was originally claimed (Mankin & Lippiello, 1971) that osteoarthritic cartilage exhibits a higher rate of synthesis of glycosaminoglycans (as gauged by ^{35}S uptake) than normal cartilage and that there is therefore an attempt at repair. Moreover, the same authors have claimed that a considerable fraction of glycosaminoglycans are turning over rapidly, so that this process of repair could be relatively fast.

Our own studies (Maroudas, 1975b; Byers et al, 1977) do not support the above results. They show that (i) sulphate incorporation is *not* increased in cartilage from osteoarthrotic joints as compared with normal cartilage and (ii) the glycosaminoglycan turn-over is so slow that any attempt at repair would be too slow to restore the tissue to its normal conditions; the turnover time for human cartilage being of the order of three years.

Of the various categories of cartilage present on the osteoarthrotic heads, it was the visually intact tissue which showed a sulphate uptake closest to that of normal cartilage when expressed on a whole wet tissue basis; on a dry basis, it had a sulphate uptake identical to that of normal cartilage. The coarsely fibrillated tissue, although having a much lower sulphate uptake when calculated on a wet basis, gave nearly the same results when the higher water content had been taken into consideration.

Increased hydration in the above tissues is thus probably one of the factors responsible for the lower cell density, as calculated on a whole tissue basis (Byers et al, 1977) and hence for a lower overall sulphate uptake. These results imply that the rate of glycosaminoglycan synthesis per cell does not show much change. It should be noted, however, that even when occasionally the presence of cell clusters was observed in the deep zone of severely fibrillated cartilage, the overall sulphate uptake was not elevated. This may be because the effect of cell necrosis was balancing or outweighing that of enhanced synthetic activity in a few cell clusters.

When sulphate incorporation is expressed per unit wieght of hexosamine, as has been done by a number of authors, higher values are obtained for severely fibrillated cartilage than for the normal tissue. It must be emphasised that this is related purely to a decrease in the glycosaminoglycan content and not to a change in the rate of glycosaminoglycan synthesis.

Acknowledgments

Table I is reproduced by permission of the publishers of Connective Tissue Research and Figure 2 by permission of the publishers of Nature.

References

Ali SY and Bayliss M (1974) In *Normal and Osteoarthritic Articular Cartilage.*
  Ed. SY Ali, MW Elves and DH Leaback, Publishers Institute of Orthopaedics, 189
Bollet AJ and Nance JL (1966) *Journal of Clinical Investigation, 45,* 1170
Bollet AJ, Handy JR and Sturgill BC (1963) *Journal of Clinical Investigation, 42,* 853
Byers PD, Maroudas A, Ostop F, Stockwell RA and Venn MF (1977) *Connective Tissue Research, 5*
Freeman M and Meachim G (1973) *Adult Articular Cartilage* Ed. MAR Freeman, Pitman Medical, London
McDevitt CA and Muir H (1976) *Journal of Bone and Joint Surgery, 58B,* 94
Mankin HJ and Lippiello L (1971) *Journal of Bone and Joint Surgery, 52A,* 424

Mankin HJ and Zarins-Thrasher (1976) *Journal of Bone and Joint Surgery, 57A,* 76
Maroudas A (1968) *Biophysical Journal, 8,* 575
Maroudas A (1970) *Biophysical Journal, 10,* 365
Maroudas A (1973) *Adult Articular Cartilage* Ed MAR Freeman, Pitman Medical,
     London, 131
Maroudas A (1975a) *Biorheology, 12,* 233
Maroudas A (1975b) *Annals of the Rheumatic Diseases, 34 suppl.2,* 55
Maroudas A (1976a) *Nature, 260,* 808
Maroudas A (1976b) *Journal of Anatomy, 122,* 335
Maroudas A and Venn MF (1977) *Annals of the Rheumatic Diseases, 36,* 399
Maroudas A, Evans H and Almeida L (1973) *Annals of the Rheumatic Diseases, 32,* 1
Mathews BF (1953) *Biochemical Journal, 96,* 710
Meachim G and Stockwell RA (1973) *Adult Articular Cartilage* Ed. MAR Freeman, Pitman
     Medical, London
Ogston AG (1970) *Chemistry and Molecular Biology of the Intercellular Matrix*
     Ed. EA Balazs, Academic Press, New York, 1231
Snowden J and Maroudas A (1976) *Biochimica Biophysica Acta, 428,* 726
Urban J (1977) *Ph.D. Thesis,* University of London
Urban J and Maroudas A (1977) In *Orthopaedic Bioengineering.* Ed. L Katz and V Mow,
     Dekker, New York. In Press
Venn MF and Maroudas A (1977) *Annals of the Rheumatic Diseases, 36,* 121

46

5

BIOCHEMICAL CHANGES IN CANINE OSTEOARTHROSIS

George Lust and Douglas R Miller

Introduction

Osteoarthrosis is a prevalent cause of degeneration of the articular cartilage, yet little is known about the fundamental determinant of this process. The casual and pathogenic relationship should be investigated in joints near the time that an abnormality is initiated. Precocious osteoarthrosis is common in canine hip dysplasia (Lust et al, 1972) and in multiple epiphysial dysplasia and familial chondrodysplasia of man (Cederbaum et al, 1976; McKusick, 1972). In this chapter we present results describing changes of collagen metabolism in osteoarthrotic cartilage of young, growing dogs. Arthrotic cartilage was obtained in a way that defined the age of lesions as about one month old.

Methods

A description of the dogs (Labrador Retrievers) used and the method of obtaining cartilage has been reported (Lust et al, 1972). Procedures used for chemical analysis, assays for metabolic and enzymatic activities and histochemical and electron microscopic analyses also have been published (Lust & Pronsky, 1972; Wiltberger & Lust, 1975). Analytical procedures for analysis of collagenous protein were done as reported (Miller & Lust, 1977 unpublished observations).

Results

The results of analyses comparing normal and degenerative articular cartilage from the hip joints of dogs have been reported (Lust & Pronsky, 1972). Studies of this type have been repeated using young, growing dogs with natural degenerative hip joint disease. Manifestations of overt disease were evident between 2.5 and seven months of age. Samples of degenerative cartilage had reproducibly less proteoglycan content, although the water content of this abnormal

47

TABLE I   Incorporation of ^{14}C-proline into Articular Cartilage Collagen and other Proteins

Fraction	Normal Cartilage	Degenerative Cartilage
	cpm/μg hypro	
Collagen (hypro)	13570	13326
Total protein (pro)	59190	77009

Samples of normal and degenerative articular cartilage were incubated with ^{14}C-proline as described in legend of Figure 1; whole cartilage was hydrolysed in 6N HCl at 110^0 for 24 hours. Aliquots of the hydrolysates were chemically analysed for hydroxyproline by the method of Switzer and Sumner (1971). Carrier hypro was added to the remainder, and the first and second toluene extracts were counted in Aquasol. The second extract (containing ^{14}C-hypro) first was passed through a column of silicic acid (0.6 x 3.2cm), reducing ^{14}C-proline to less than 0.5% of counts initially present. Both proline and hydroxyproline counts are expressed per μg hydroxyproline.

tissue was increased from 5–8%. DNA content per mg cartilage did not change significantly. In vitro incubations of normal and degenerative cartilage dices with thymidine–^{14}CH$_3$ and with Na$_2$^{35}SO$_4$ resulted in reduced incorporation of the radioactive precursor into DNA and proteoglycan of degenerative cartilage. Specific radioactivities (cpm/μg) indicated that the turnover of proteoglycans was slightly increased, whereas that of DNA was lower in degenerative samples (Lust et al, 1972).

Results of electron microscopic studies of canine articular cartilage have been reported (Wiltberger & Lust, 1975). Ultrastructural changes in degenerative cartilage were prominent in the upper 0.5mm of cartilage. It was found that the tightly packed collagen fibrils of the surface layer were absent in lesions. An amorphous material was found near the uneven, fissured surface. Below the surface layer the proportion of large collagen fibrils was less in lesions than in normal cartilage, and the overall number of fibrils per μm^2 in degenerative cartilage increased with depth into the tissue. The oblong cells of the upper layer of normal cartilage were not found in the degenerative samples; however other differences between cells in deeper normal and abnormal cartilage were minimal. Although not established unequivocally, these results suggested that the surface of articular cartilage was the place of initial insult.

The content of collagen (total hydroxyproline per mg cartilage), was not changed significantly when normal and osteoarthrotic cartilage was analysed. Collagen synthesis was measured by determining the rate of conversion of C^{14} proline to C^{14} hydroxyproline (see Table I). An increased rate of incorporation of C^{14} proline into recently synthesised proteins of degenerative cartilage was observed. However, the apparent rate of collagen synthesis was the same in normal and osteoarthrotic cartilage, since the specific activities (cpm/μg) of hydroxyproline in the two kinds of tissue were similar.

Analysis of cartilage extracts using SDS polyacrylamide gel electrophoresis

SDS-PAGE Patterns

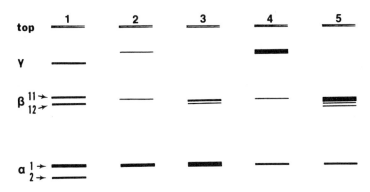

Figure 1   Electrophoretic patterns of collagen obtained from extracts of normal and
degenerative articular cartilage. Samples of normal and degenerative cartilage (100mg)
were incubated in 3 ml of Dulbecco's Modified Eagle Medium containing 10% fetal
calf serum, 50 μg/ml ascorbic acid, 300 μg/ml glutamine, 100 μg/ml β-aminopropioni-
trile, 30 μg/ml α ketoglutarate, 20 units/ml pen-strep, and 20 μCi/ml C^{14} proline in
an atmosphere of 10% CO_2 – 90% air for 24 hours at 37°C. Samples then were
washed three times in 0.9% saline and placed into 0.01 M phosphate buffer, pH 7.5,
containing 0.2% SDS, 2 M urea, and 1% sucrose in a ratio of 100 mg cartilage/ml, and
heated for 1/2 hour at 65°C. When reducing conditions were desired this buffer
contained in addition 2% 2-mercaptoethanol (2–ME). Cartilage then was diced,
allowed to stand overnight at room temperature, and reheated for 1/2 hour prior to
application to the gels. Twenty-five μl aliquots were applied to 4% polyacrylamide
gels, 10 cm in length, and electrophoresed for six hours using a current of 6mA/gel.
A sample of calf skin collagen (Sigma) was run with each set of gels for comparative
purposes. Gels were fixed and stained in 50% methanol, 5% acetic acid, 0.2% Coomassie
blue for two hours, and destained in a commercial diffusion apparatus in 10% methanol,
5% acetic acid. 1 – Calf skin collagen standard. 2 – Normal cartilage extract.
3 – Normal cartilage extract, with 2% 2–ME. 4 – Degenerative cartilage extracts.
5 – Degenerative cartilage extract, with 2% 2–ME.

revealed differences in the kind of collagenous proteins present in normal and
degenerative cartilage. The electrophoretic analysis suggested that degenerative
cartilage contained increased amounts of a high molecular weight species which
was not prominent in extracts of normal samples. Its molecular weight was
estimated to be greater than 300,000 daltons (γ collagen chains of calf skin
and dog skin standard were about 300,000 daltons). The accumulated high
molecular weight material was not found in the same location after reduction
with 2–mercaptoethanol (see Figure 1, gel nos. 4 and 5).

SDS-agarose gel filtration (column of Sepharose 6B 1.5 x 95 cm) substanti-
ated the presence of a high molecular weight collagenous protein in degenerative
cartilage. Its molecular weight was estimated to be about 450,000 daltons. In
normal tissue this material was found in much smaller amounts. Reduction of
the high molecular weight collagenous protein with 2–mercaptoethanol
eliminated the peak with a MW of about 450,000 daltons (Figure 2). Treatment

49

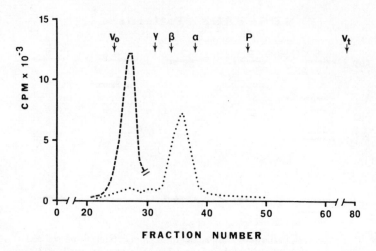

Figure 2   Collagen–C^{14} (^{14}C-hydroxyproline) profiles from degenerative cartilage extract
eluted without 2–ME (- - -) and with 2–ME (. . . .). 100 mg of degenerative cartilage
was incubated, and extracted as described in Figure 1. Two ml of the extract was
applied to a column of Sepharose 6B (Pharmacia) (1.5 x 95 cm). Elution of collagenous
proteins was with 0.1% SDS in 0.01 M phosphate buffer, pH 7.5 using a flow rate of
approximately 5 ml/hr. Two μCi of ^{3}H-glycine was added to measure the total volume
(V_T) of the column for each run. 2.0 ml fractions were collected, lyophilised,
hydrolysed in six N HCl at 110°C for 24 hours, and analysed for ^{14}C-hydroxyproline,
after addition of carrier hydroxyproline, by the method of Switzer and Sumner (1971).
Fractions 20–30 were pooled, reduced by the addition of 2-mercaptoethanol to a
concentration of 2%, and rechromatographed on the same column using the above
buffer containing 0.1% 2–ME. Arrows above the profiles indicate the elution points
of column calibration standards: void volume (V_o), determined using blue dextran
2000; γ chains of canine articular cartilage collagen ($\sim$ 300,000 daltons); β collagen
chains ($\sim$ 200,000 daltons); α collagen chains ($\sim$ 100,000 daltons); and pepsin (P)
(35,000 daltons). A plot of V_E/V_T versus log MW was linear.

of the cartilage with 0.1% pepsin at pH3 for 18 hours at 4°C resulted in the
total disappearance of the high MW material in Figure 2. It was concluded that
this collagenous protein was a procollagen of articular cartilage.

Discussion

The basic cause of osteoarthrosis is unknown. The data reported in this paper
suggest that a defect in the conversion of procollagen to collagen may have a
role in this in canine articular cartilage. It remains to be elucidated whether
this abnormality is involved in the initiation of degeneration of cartilage or
whether its effect is in the progression of the disease state.

Comparison of cartilage extracts by SDS gel electrophoresis showed that
extracts from degenerative cartilage contained increased amounts of high
molecular weight collagens. The majority of this was sensitive to limited
pepsin digestion, resulting in the same electrophoretic pattern as the normal
cartilage. Chromatographic analysis of extracts on 6% agarose columns

indicated that the degenerative samples contained a collagenous protein with a molecular weight of about 450,000 daltons which was reducible with 2-mercaptoethanol to one of 150,000 daltons. These results supported the concept that the high molecular weight collagenous protein was procollagen.

The mechanisms for the increased procollagen content are under study now. Increased synthesis of procollagen, decreased activity of procollagen peptidase, and removal, inhibition or destruction of this enzyme, are possibilities. Procollagen peptidase deficiency was not complete since a portion of the collagen in degenerative cartilage apparently was processed normally. Cattle and sheep (Lapiere et al, 1971) affected with dermatosporaxis, and humans with Ehrlers-Danlos syndrome type VII (Lichtenstein et al, 1973), have defects in procollagen peptidase. Decreased organisation and size of collagen fibrils in tissues affected by these diseases were reported and resemble ultrastructural observations made on degenerative cartilage (Wiltberger & Lust, 1975).

More research is needed to answer questions concerned with cartilage degeneration. The interplay of collagen metabolism and structure with proteoglycans requires additional study. It appears likely that factors such as joint conformation, weight bearing stresses, and the involvement of tissue activating compounds or immunological reactions may be required as aggravating stimuli to cause a partial defect in collagen processing.

Acknowledgments

Research was supported by the John M Olin Foundation and the Richard King Mellon Foundation.

References

Cederbaum SD, Kaitila I, Rimoin DL, Stiehm ER, (1976) *The Journal of Pediatrics, 89,* 737
Lapiere CM, Lenaers A, Kohn LD, (1971) *Proceedings of the National Academy of Sciences (USA), 68,* 3054
Lichtenstein JR, Martins GR, Kohn LD, Byers PH, McKusick VA, (1973) *Science, 182,* 298
Lust G, Farrell PW, Sheffy BE, (1977) *ARC Workshop Models for Osteoarthrosis.* Ed G Nuki, Pitman Medical, Tunbridge Wells
Lust G, Pronsky W, Sherman DM, (1972) *American Journal of Veterinary Research, 33,* 2429
Lust G and Pronsky W, (1972) *Clinica Chimica Acta, 39,* 281
McKusick VA, (1972) In *Arthritis and Allied Conditions.* Eds JL Hollander and DJ McCarty, 8th Edition, Philadelphia, Lea and Febiger, p.1340
Switzer BE and Sumner GF, (1971) *Analytical Biochemistry, 39,* 487
Wiltberger H and Lust G, (1975) *American Journal of Veterinary Research, 36,* 727

6

MACROMOLECULAR BIOCHEMISTRY OF CARTILAGE IN THE INITIAL STAGES OF EXPERIMENTAL CANINE OSTEOARTHROSIS

Cahir McDevitt, Helen Muir and David Eyre

Introduction

There is considerable evidence to suggest that cartilage is affected in the early stages of osteoarthrosis and hence the biomechanical function of collagen and proteoglycans, the two most important constituents of cartilage, have received considerable attention. In human cartilage the tensile properties are closely correlated with the collagen content (Kempson et al, 1973) whereas compressive stiffness shows very good correlation with total glycosaminoglycan content (Kempson et al, 1970). These and other studies (Maroudas et al, 1969; Bjelle, 1975) also show that there is considerable variation in the topographical distribution of collagen, chondroitin sulphate and keratan sulphate in cartilage from different areas of the same joint and between different individuals irrespective of age or sex. In studies of osteoarthrosis this fact presents problems in choosing appropriate controls.

To study the initial stages of the disease process, a suitable model has to be selected that (1) reproduces the natural disease as closely as possible with the minimum of manipulation, (2) uses a species in which growth and remodelling have ceased at the time the experiments are done, (3) involves joints of sufficient size to enable samples of cartilage to be taken from different areas of the joint surface for biochemical analysis and (4) provides appropriate controls.

We have found that the dog meets all these requirements and as we have developed micromethods for the qualitative assessment of macromolecules, the size of the joint is sufficient to enable cartilage from different areas of the same joint to be sampled.

Experimental Design

Mature dogs of various breeds, 15–30kg in weight and of both sexes, were used. Skeletal maturity and absence of osteoarthrosis were established by clinical and

Medial   Lateral

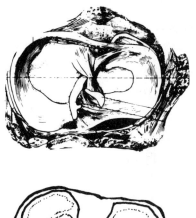

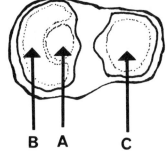

B   A   C

Figure 1   Areas of tibia sampled

radiological examination. The anterior cruciate ligament of one knee was cut by
a 2mm stab incision into the joint, the other knee serving as a control (Gilbertson,
1975). The dogs were exercised for half to one hour each day and killed at
intervals from 1–48 weeks after the operation. In sham operations a stab incision
was made but the ligament left intact. The articular cartilage of the tibia, femur
and patella of control and operated joints were removed and kept separately. The
tibial cartilage was divided into three areas (Figure 1) and each examined separately
(McDevitt & Muir, 1976). The lesions invariably developed in area A of the tibia.
    This experimental model of osteoarthrosis has the following advantages.
(a) The procedure is analogous to a natural cause of 'secondary' osteoarthrosis in
dogs (Tirgari & Vaughan, 1975) due to instability of the knee resulting from
accidental rupture of the anterior cruciate ligament; (b) the joint is not exposed;
(c) no foreign matter is introduced; (d) the time of onset is known exactly; (e)
the lesion appears in the same region of the tibial surface in every dog, which
enables this area to be sampled *before* lesions have developed. This requirement
is essential if the initial events in the disease process are to be studied.

Pathological Assessment

Before dissection of the cartilage from the bone, the quality of the articular surface was graded visually as described by Meachim (1972) by the penetration of indian ink. No ink penetrated the intact surface (Grade 1), when there was minimal fibrillation, specks or grey patches were seen (Grade 2) and dark patches were produced when there was overt fibrillation (Grade 3).

Sagittal sections of cartilage from three sites on the tibia (Figure 1) and from femur and patella were taken for histology and stained with Saffranin O (Rosenberg 1971) and haematoxylin-eosin.

Calcified and decalcified vertical sections of femurs from experimental, control and sham operated joints were also prepared for histology (Gilbertson, 1975).

The changes observed in cartilage and bone in operated joints were progressive

TABLE I   Histology of Sagittal Sections of Tibial, Femoral and Patellar Cartilage at Different times after Ligament Section (McDevitt et al, 1977)

	Weeks after operation	Tibia			Femoral condyle	Patella
		A	B	C		
Experimental osteoarthritis						
Articular surface	1	+	−	−	+	−
Loss of Safranin O		−	−	−	−	−
Cell clones		+	+	+	+	+
Articular surface	2	++	−	+	++	−
Loss of Safranin O		−	−	−	−	−
Cell clones		++	++	++	++	++
Articular surface	7	+++	−	+	++	−
Loss of Safranin O		−	−	−	−	−
Cell clones		++	++	++	++	++
Articular surface	16	++++	++	++	+++	++
Loss of Safranin O		+	−	−	+	−
Cell clones		+++	++	++	+++	++
Natural osteoarthritis						
(Dog-Y)						
Articular surface		++++	++	++	++++	++
Loss of Safranin O		+	−	−	+	++
Cell clones		+++	++	++	+++	++

Key to Scores
Quality of articular surface: − intact surface; + slight roughening; ++ roughening and small clefts; +++ roughening and fissures to middle zone; ++++ total disruption of surface layer.
Loss of Safranin O: − no loss of Safranin O staining; + decreased Safranin O staining in superficial zone.
Cell clones: + increased cell density; ++ occasional cell 'doublets'; +++ clones of two or more cells evident.

54

TABLE II. Similarity of Natural and Experimental Canine Osteoarthrosis of the Knee

CARTILAGE	(1)	Location of lesions	
	(2)	Macroscopical appearance of lesions	
	(3)	Histology	
	(4)	Progression in severity	
	(5)	Biochemical changes in cartilage	
		Cartilage	softens and holds more water
		Proteoglycans	more extractable composition changes aggregation reduced
BONE		Osteophytes	
MENISCUS		Rupture of medial meniscus	
SYNOVIAL MEMBRANE		Discolouration and vascular proliferation	

(Table I) (McDevitt et al, 1977) and became indistinguishable from those of natural osteoarthrosis (Table II), but were not seen in sham operated joints.

Overall Analysis of Cartilage

Representative samples of whole cartilage from the different areas of the joint surface were analysed for contents of water, collagen, chondroitin sulphate (uronic acid) and 'keratan sulphate' (from ratio of glucosamine/galactosamine in relation to uronic acid) (McDevitt & Muir, 1975, 1976). Cartilage near the edge of the joint surface was not used, and care was taken in the dissection to avoid tissue from the osteo-chondral junction as assessed by histology.

Water Content

The earliest change was an increase in water content in area A of the tibia which later spread to surrounding areas of the tibia and to the femur and patella. The increase on average was about 6—8% (Figure 2). There was no change in water content in sham operated joints and by the time lesions were well developed in area A, the water content decreased slightly below the levels for corresponding areas of the control joint.

The increase in water content was a very early change that soon affected the entire cartilage of the joint, even those areas where lesions did not develop.

Chondroitin Sulphate Content

Since chondroitin sulphate contains galactosamine and uronic acid whereas keratan sulphate contains glucosamine and galactose, the molar ratio of galactosamine to glucosamine together with the uronic acid content of the cartilage

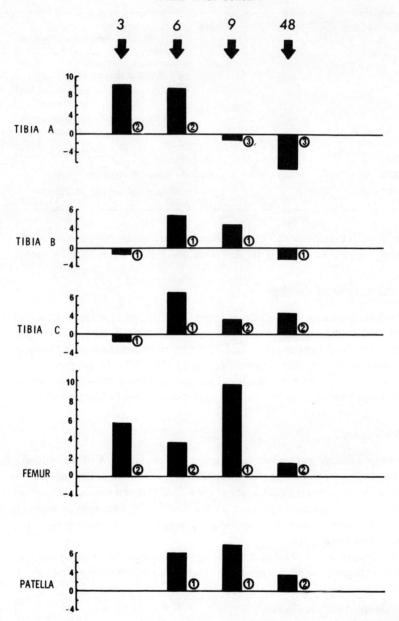

WEEKS AFTER SURGERY

Figure 2. Differences in water content of tibial cartilage from three areas shown in Figure 1 of operated and control joints. The scales (not all equal) show per cent differences from controls

56

provides an approximate estimate of the keratan sulphate content of the tissue. This decreased in all samples of cartilage from operated joints. The actual molar ratios varied considerably between one animal and another and hence it was imperative to use as a control the cartilage from the unoperated knee of the same animal (McDevitt & Muir, 1976).

The increase in galactosamine/glucosamine molar ratios began at about the same time as the increase in water content and was more pronounced in extracted proteoglycans than in those remaining in the tissue. Again this change was first evident in area A of the tibia and subsequently affected areas B and C, as well as the patella and femur.

Proteoglycans

Dissociating solvents such as 2M $CaCl_2$ or 4M guanidine HCl are effective in extracting proteoglycans from cartilage (Sajdera & Hascall, 1969). The cartilage specimens were extracted by a standard procedure using 2M $CaCl_2$ (McDevitt & Muir, 1975, 1976). As a consequence of the increase in hydration and loosening of the collagen network, the proteoglycans became progressively easier to extract by a standard procedure using 2M $CaCl_2$ so that from areas having grade 3 lesions, 70–90% was extracted compared with about 50% from control cartilage. Again this change affected area A of the tibia before the other two areas (Figure 3). There was no equivalent increase in the proportion of the total non-collagenous protein extracted (McDevitt et al, 1973).

Purification of Proteoglycans and Dissociation of Proteoglycan Aggregates

When dialysed to low ionic strength, a proportion of the proteoglycan extracted with dissociating solvents re-associates into aggregates which appear as a fast sedimenting component in the analytical ultracentrifuge (Hascall & Sajdera, 1969). Proteoglycans may be purified from contaminating proteins by caesium chloride density gradient centrifugation. In this method molecules are separated according to their buoyant density in a concentrated caesium chloride gradient. Proteoglycans have a high buoyant density in caesium chloride and hence separate at the bottom of the gradient whilst contaminating proteins that are not bound to proteoglycan separate at the top. Purified aggregated and non-aggregated proteoglycans are thus obtained from the bottom of the caesium chloride gradient. Aggregates are not dissociated under these conditions and hence this is referred to as 'associative' density gradient centrifugation (Figure 4).

Under 'dissociative' conditions when 4M guanidine HCl is added to the caesium chloride, aggregated proteoglycans are dissociated and the constituents of the aggregates are separated from each other, with dissociated proteoglycans

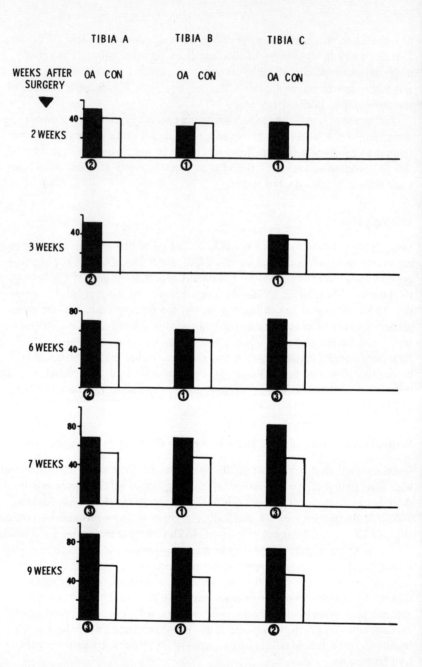

Figure 3. Comparison of the relative amounts of proteoglycans extracted by 2M CaCl$_2$ pH 6.8 from osteoarthrotic and control cartilage, expressed as a percentage of the total uronic acid in the tissue. Areas of tibial cartilage samples shown in Figure 1

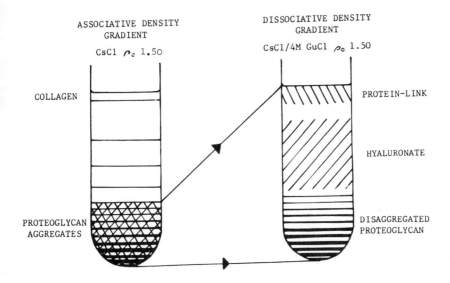

ASSOCIATIVE DENSITY GRADIENT

CsCl ρ_c 1.50

DISSOCIATIVE DENSITY GRADIENT

CsCl/4M GuCl ρ_c 1.50

COLLAGEN

PROTEOGLYCAN AGGREGATES

PROTEIN-LINK

HYALURONATE

DISAGGREGATED PROTEOGLYCAN

Figure 4. Equilibrium density gradient centrifugation in caesium chloride of proteoglycans of articular cartilage.
A. *Associative Conditions* Starting density 1.5 g/ml centrifuged at 100,000 g_{av} for 48h at 20°C.
B. *Dissociative Conditions* Lower fraction from associative gradient mixed with an equal volume of 7.5M guanidinium chloride at pH 5.8. Starting density adjusted to 1.5 g/ml with caesium chloride

at the bottom of the gradient, hyaluronic acid in the middle and the third constituent, the link-protein at the top (Figure 4) (Hardingham & Muir, 1974; Hascall & Heinegard, 1974).

The proteoglycans extracted from the cartilage samples were each separately submitted to 'associative' and 'dissociative' density gradient centrifugation employing somewhat lower starting densities than those employed originally by Hascall and Sajdera (1969) for use with proteoglycans from nasal cartilage.

Results

I. Quality of Proteoglycans

Composition Purified proteoglycans were analysed for uronic acid and protein content and the relative proportion of chondroitin sulphate to keratan sulphate determined from molar ratios of galactosamine to glucosamine after hydrolysis. After dissociative density gradient centrifugation proteoglycans extracted from each of the cartilages of operated joints invariably had a higher proportion of chondroitin sulphate relative to keratan sulphate than did proteoglycans extracted from corresponding control cartilages.

Molecular size of purified proteoglycans was compared by gel chromatography on Sepharose 2B, analytical ultracentrifugation and gel electrophoresis.

a) Proteoglycans Prepared Under 'Associative' Conditions

The proportion of the total proteoglycans that were large enough to be excluded from Sepharose 2B did not change for several months after the operation, but in the analytical ultracentrifuge, the fast sedimenting proteoglycan aggregates became more heterogeneous with time after the operation.

Preparative gel chromatography on Sepharose 2B was used to prepare four proteoglycan fractions of decreasing molecular size from control and experimental cartilage 48 weeks after the operation. Although the range of molecular size was unchanged the molar ratio of galactosamine to glucosamine had increased in all four fractions, particularly in the largest included fraction (Kav 0.33) (Table III). The weight ratio of uronic acid to protein had also increased appreciably, particularly in this fraction, but also in the other three (Table III). This

TABLE III. Chemical Composition of Proteoglycans Extracted from Tibial Cartilage of Control and Experimental Joints 48 Weeks after Operation. Proteoglycans were Purified by Density Gradient Centrifugation under 'Associative' Conditions and Chromatographed on Sepharose 2B. Fractions were Obtained in Order of Elution Beginning with the Excluded Fraction ($K_{av}=0$)

K_{av}	Molar Ratio Galactosamine/Glucosamine		Weight Ratio Uronate/Protein	
	OA	CON	OA	CON
0	1.93	1.66	1.13	1.04
0.33	4.63	3.60	3.52	2.85
0.46	3.83	3.43	2.93	2.88
0.63	2.34	1.75	1.69	1.55

indicates that at 48 weeks when grade 3 lesions had developed, the proteoglycans were not degraded and reduced in size but that proteoglycans of a different composition had been formed containing a higher proportion of chondroitin sulphate.

b) Proteoglycans Prepared Under 'Dissociative' Conditions

The gel chromatographic profile of dissociated proteoglycans changed little even six months after the operation and there was no increase in the degree of polydispersity.

II. Quality of Newly Synthesised Proteoglycans

Proteoglycans labelled in vivo with $^{35}SO_4$ were isolated from control and experimental cartilage at various times up to ten weeks after the operation. The isotopes were injected into the joint space and the dogs killed four days or eight days later.

The newly formed proteoglycans, isolated and purified as before, were examined by gel chromatography on micro-Sepharose 2B columns, and the elution profile of labelled material determined.

Labelled proteoglycan prepared under associative conditions showed the same elution profile from control and experimental cartilage. The labelled proteoglycans were also prepared under dissociative conditions and gave similar gel chromatographic profiles.

The ability of dissociative labelled proteoglycans to interact with hyaluronate was assessed on gel-chromatography by comparing the elution profile of labelled material before and after the addition of 1% by weight of hyaluronate (Hardingham & Muir, 1972). The newly formed proteoglycans in control and experimental cartilage, including all three areas of tibial cartilage interacted with hyaluronate to an equal extent, even when the proteoglycans had been extracted from areas of cartilage where lesions had developed.

Total, as well as labelled proteoglycans from control and experimental cartilage were also compared on dissociative density gradient centrifugation. The cartilage was taken from each of the three areas of the tibia of two dogs ten weeks after the operation. Labelled proteoglycans distributed in the gradient in the same way as the total unlabelled proteoglycans in control and experimental samples, even when grade 3 lesions had developed in area A and grade 2 lesions in areas B and C. All fractions of proteoglycans from experimental tissue had higher galactosamine/glucosamine molar ratios than corresponding fractions from control cartilage. This change was particularly marked in the fractions of highest buoyant density which contain no hyaluronate and which represent the majority of the total proteoglycan (Hardingham & Muir, 1974).

III. Collagen

Cartilage contains type II collagen (Miller & Matukas, 1974) which accounts for the major proportion of the dry weight of articular cartilage. Collagen synthesis was examined in vivo using ^{3}H-proline given by intra-articular injection (Eyre et al, 1975). Dogs were killed 2, 8 and 24 weeks after ligament resection. Synthesis of collagen was measured by the formation of labelled hydroxyproline and total protein synthesis by the incorporation of label into protein. The type of collagen synthesised was established by the isolation and quantitation of specific labelled peptides produced by cyanogen bromide cleavage (Eyre & Muir, 1974).

After extraction of proteoglycans the relative proportion of newly formed collagen and total protein synthesised in the cartilage residue was compared in

61

TABLE IV. Collagen Synthesis Relative to Total Protein Synthesis (After Extraction of Proteoglycans)

Weeks after Surgery	% Total Protein Synthesis (Pooled Tissue)	
	Control	OA
2	5	27
8	5	33
24	18	41

the cartilage of control and operated joints. In the former, collagen synthesis accounted for only a few percent of total protein synthesis, whereas in operated joints it accounted for increasing proportions as the disease progressed (Table IV).

The labelled CNBr cleavage peptides Co-chromatographed with the peptides

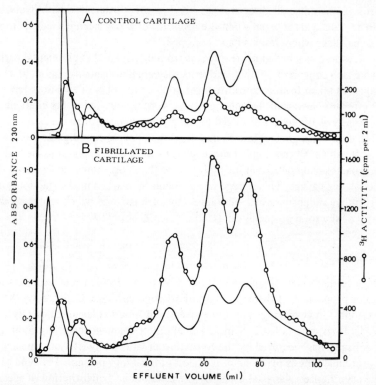

Figure 5. Chromatography on CM-cellulose of CNBr-peptides of collagen from dog articular cartilage labelled in vivo with ^{3}H proline. 10—15mg of each digest was eluted from the column (0.9cm x 6cm) at 42°C with a linear gradient of NaCl (0.02—0.15mol/L) in a total volume of 150ml of 0.02mol/L Na citrate-citric acid, pH 3.6. (From Eyre et al, 1975)

of type II collagen of control and operated joints (Figure 5) and hence at this stage of the disease process when grade 2 and grade 3 lesions had developed no type I collagen was detected by these procedures.

It is concluded that synthesis of collagen increases during the development of experimental osteoarthrosis but that the normal type II collagen is produced and laid down in the matrix.

Conclusions

In the early stages of the experimental disease studied here, although the proteoglycans had changed in composition, their range of molecular size had not. They were therefore not degraded. This conclusion is supported by the finding that

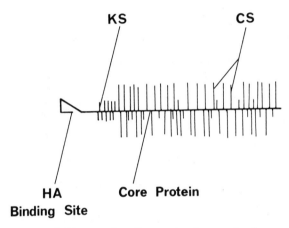

Figure 6. Diagram of cartilage proteoglycan molecule

newly formed proteoglycans in control and experimental cartilages were equally able to interact with hyaluronate and hence the hyaluronate binding region was intact (Figure 6) even though it is very sensitive to chemical modification (Hardingham et al, 1976) and proteolytic degradation. However, analytical ultracentrifugation showed the aggregated proteoglycans from experimental cartilage to be heterogeneous, which suggests that some alteration in hyaluronate may have occurred.

General Conclusions

In experimental and natural osteoarthrosis there is an increase in hydration and proteoglycans are formed that are qualitatively different from those in normal cartilage. In experimental osteoarthrosis the biochemical changes preceded the

63

appearance of lesions and these were at first localised to the regions of greatest stress where lesions subsequently developed. The surrounding areas were thereafter affected and finally the entire cartilage of the joint was involved even in regions where lesions did not develop, but there was no evidence that the proteoglycans of the tissue were degraded.

Acknowledgments

Table I is reproduced by the publishers of the Journal of Bone and Joint Surgery and Figure 5 by permission of the publishers of the Annals of the Rheumatic Diseases.

References

Bjelle, A (1975) *Connective Tissue Research, 3,* 141

Eyre, DR and Muir, H (1974) *FEBS Letters, 42,* 192

Eyre, DR, McDevitt, CA and Muir, H (1975) *Annals of the Rheumatic Diseases, 34, Suppt.2,* 137

Gilbertson, EMM (1975) *Annals of the Rheumatic Diseases, 34,* 12

Hardingham, TE and Muir, H (1972) *Biochimica et Biophysica Acta, 279,* 401

Hardingham, TE and Muir, H (1974) *Biochemical Journal, 139,* 565

Hardingham, TE, Ewins, RJF and Muir, H (1976) *Biochemical Journal, 157,* 127

Hascall, VC and Heinegard, D (1974) *Journal of Biological Chemistry, 249,* 4232

Hascall, VC and Sajdera, SW (1969) *Journal of Biological Chemistry, 244,* 2384

Kempson, GE, Muir, H, Swanson, SAV and Freeman, MAR (1970) *Biochimica et Biophysica Acta, 215,* 70

Kempson, GE, Muir, H, Pollard, C and Tuke, M (1973) *Biochimica et Biophysica Acta, 297,* 465

Maroudas, A, Muir, H and Wingham, J (1969) *Biochemica et Biophysica Acta, 177,* 492

McDevitt, CA and Muir, H (1975) In *Protides of Biological Fluids.* (Ed) J Peeters. Pergamon Press, Oxford. Page 269

McDevitt, CA and Muir, H (1976) *Journal of Bone and Joint Surgery, 58B,* 94

McDevitt, CA, Gilbertson, EMM and Muir, H (1977) *Journal of Bone and Joint Surgery, 59B,* 24

McDevitt, CA, Muir, H and Pond, MJ (1973) *Biochemical Society Transactions, 1,* 287

Meachim, G (1972) *Annals of the Rheumatic Diseases, 31,* 457

Miller, EJ and Matukas, VJ (1974) *Federation Proceedings of American Societies for Experimental Biology, 33,* 197

Rosenberg, L (1971) *Journal of Bone and Joint Surgery, 53A,* 69

Sajdera, SW and Hascall, VC (1969) *Journal of Biological Chemistry, 244,* 77

Tirgari, M and Vaughan, LC (1975) *Veterinary Record, 96,* 394

7

THE RELATIONSHIP BETWEEN AGE, THICKNESS, SURFACE STRUCTURE, COMPLIANCE AND COMPOSITION OF HUMAN FEMORAL HEAD ARTICULAR CARTILAGE

D L Gardner, R J Elliott, C G Armstrong and R B Longmore

All mammals are subject to a common disorder of diarthrodial joints that causes great disability as a result of cartilage loss and the remodelling of nearby bone. This disorder, osteoarthrosis (OA) (Gardner, 1972a) can be the end result of any hereditary or environmental disease that significantly disturbs the structure and function of hyaline articular cartilage. However, in the majority of instances in man, in whom this disorder causes clinical signs and symptoms, the closest analysis fails to reveal any single identifiable explanation for the disabling illness.

The causes of OA have been sought, for more than 70 years, with increasing vigour and with the application of devices of ever-increasing technical sophistication. There are many theories to account for the onset of OA. Not all are mutually exclusive.

Genetic factors may be implicated. In the uncommon generalised form of OA the systemic illness and the sequential involvement of series of synovial joints, including the distal interphalangeal, is familial in nature and involves a genetic factor that is not well understood but is not indexed by HLA marker gene loci. OA is less evident in those who have osteoporosis than in persons with normal bone structure. Increasing numbers of microfractures in subchondral bone may lead to a failure of this material and a consequent secondary failure of cartilage (Radin, 1974). As a material, cartilage may fail as an aggregate or because of disorganisation of one of its main components. In this sense, attention has been mainly directed to collagen (Freeman, 1975; Weightman, 1976). However, with age the elastic response of articular hyaline cartilage to loading forces decreases with decreasing content of glycosaminoglycan (GAG) (Kempson et al, 1970). This evidence and the more recent demonstration that there is a diminishing content of proteoglycan (PG) aggregates with age (Brandt & Palmoski, 1976), strongly suggest that changes in the PG macromolecules, which are intimately associated with collagen in vivo, may also lead to mechanical failure of cartilage as a load-bearing material. It has proved exceedingly difficult to dissociate concepts of the origin of OA from views that emphasise the critical role of the highly efficient lubricant, synovial fluid, in joint function. Contemporary theories stress the importance of boundary lubrication (Mow et al, 1974) and show how lubrication mechanisms change at different phases of common movements such as walking (Unsworth et al, 1975). These theories draw attention to failure of the lubricating mechanism rather than of the bearing surfaces. That there is an enzymatic, metabolic or inflammatory origin for OA finds little support in spite of the high frequency of secondary OA in common diseases such as rheumatoid arthritis. That a primary release of proteolytic enzymes from synovial cells can degrade cartilage surfaces (Glynn, 1977) is of uncertain significance. The experimental observation that prostaglandin A_1 can injure or kill chondrocytes in vitro (Kirkpatrick & Gardner, 1977) is equally of unknown relevance. Neuronal diseases can lead rapidly to OA in the rare tabetic and syringomyelic neurogenic arthropathies, and experimentally, in diarthrodial joints deprived of their afferent sensory innervation. It cannot be argued that loss of protective neuro-muscular reflexes play any part in the commonplace forms of OA. Similarly endocrine diseases, such as myxoedema and acromegaly, can precipitate unusual forms of OA but it is not accepted that endocrine factors lead to the common form of the disorder.

The central theme running through these theories remains the importance of hyaline cartilage itself. A full understanding of the molecular composition, gross structure and physical properties of cartilage is a pre-requisite for a reasonable assessment of the aetiopathogenesis of OA. Critical questions remain unanswered: What is the mass, volume, extent and thickness of articular cartilage in joints that are often severely affected by OA?   What are the relationships between these variables and factors such as age, sex, body weight, height, mechanical stresses and occupation?   How do these variables relate to changes in the mechanical properties of cartilage?

There are no published measurements of the mass and volume of the cartilage of normal adult human hip joints. The thickness of femoral head cartilage has now been recorded in detail by Armstrong (1976) and by Armstrong and Gardner (1977). There are few comparable reports. Kempson (1973) gave thickness measurements for a limited number of specimens. Meachim (1971) derived data for cartilage thickness for the human shoulder joint and Simon et al (1973) measured the thickness of animal synovial joint cartilage.

The present investigations derive from these questions. They examine the surface structure, thickness and mechanical properties of femoral head cartilage and relate these variables to preliminary measurements of the GAG content of cartilage at different ages. In the course of this work the validity of earlier studies (Kempson, 1973; Radin, 1974; Sokoloff, 1968; Woo et al, 1976) on the mechanical properties of cartilage has been questioned. In previous studies, mechanical tests have often been limited to parts of disarticulated joint surfaces. The tests have frequently been made with indentors or plates of small relative area. The loads applied have borne little relationship to those now known to occur in joints during life. For these reasons anomalous estimates have been obtained of the physical properties of the whole organised material as it is likely to exist in vivo.

Our results are presented in four parts. First, we describe the emergence of present views on the three-dimensional surface structure of cartilage. Second, we analyse measurements of femoral head cartilage thickness, relating these measurements to age in 28 subjects. Third, in a further series of normal subjects, the response of loading tests of 28 whole hip joints is given, enabling the deformability of ageing cartilage to be derived. Finally, preliminary measurements are described of the chemical composition of human lateral femoral condylar cartilage. These results are contrasted with those from the optical and mechanical measurements and used to formulate an hypothesis to explain the origin and progression of osteoarthrosis.

Articular cartilage surface structure
(Gardner, 1972b; Longmore & Gardner, 1975; Longmore, 1976; Longmore & Gardner, 1977 unpublished observations.)

Historically, load-bearing, hyaline articular cartilage surfaces, including those of the hip joint, were assumed to be 'conspicuously smooth' (Davies, 1969) (Figure 1). Since 1968, it has come to be accepted that in the non-loaded in

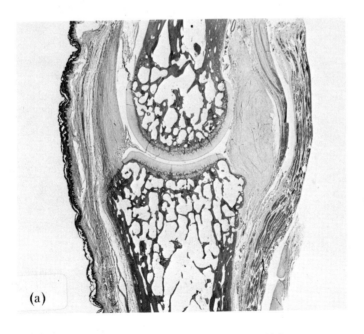

(a)

Figure 1   Longitudinal section through a normal adult synovial joint

67

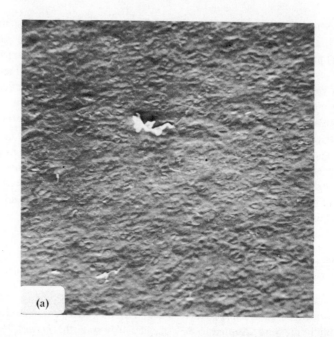

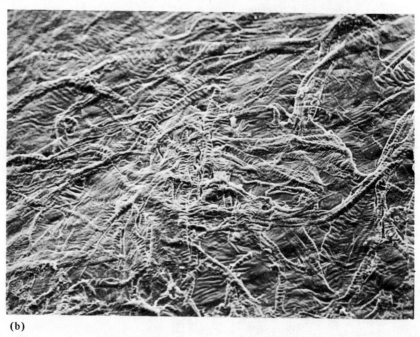

Figure 2   Scanning electron micrographs of the surface of human femoral condyle.
a) infant (x 200); b) 45 year old adult (x 140)

vitro condition, when the surfaces are freed from synovial fluid, this is not correct (Dowson et al, 1968; Gardner & Woodward, 1968; McCall, 1968; Inoue et al, 1968). Evidence has accumulated that the normal surfaces are covered by a large series of 20–40 μm hollows (Figure 2a, b) superimposed on the broad primary anatomical contours and the secondary 0.5 mm irregularities detectable with a hand lens. The location of tertiary hollows probably corresponds to the most superficial chondrocytes that lie 1–5 μm beneath the load-bearing surface (Clarke, 1972). It is possible that the hollows persist under sustained loads during periods in which the anatomical contours deform reversibly by the loss and subsequent intake of water.

Whether the tertiary hollows retain lubricant and indirectly 'boost' lubrication (Dowson et al, 1968) is doubted. They are present on the surfaces of foetal diarthrodial joints, the fibrocartilage of knee joint menisci and the temperomandibular fibrocartilagenous discs. They are neither artefactual nor acquired by use i.e. in response to repeated abnormal movements and loads.

For some years it has appeared that the ratio of cartilage matrix volume chondrocyte count increases with age (Stockwell & Meachim, 1973). Since the chondrocytes at articular surfaces reflect the sites of surface tertiary hollows, it was logical to ask whether these hollows changed in frequency and in size with age. Using the Leitz reflected light interference microscope (RLIM), Longmore (1976) studied the surfaces of the lateral femoral condyles removed at necropsy from 20 normal subjects aged 0–47 years. The mean age was 19.25 years. In the normal reflected light mode, the RLIM provided a precise view of the surfaces freed from synovial fluid. In the interference mode, using a narrow band width of green light (λ = 550 nm), a discrete pattern of surface contours was revealed (Gardner & Longmore, 1974) (Figure 3). The diameter of the hollows, their depth and their frequency were ascertained and statistical analyses conducted to determine whether these variables changed with age. The results (Longmore & Gardner, 1975) revealed that there was a decrease in hollow frequency with age (Figure 4); that the depth of the hollows increased with age from 0.6 – 0.7 μm at age 0–5 years to 1.4–1.7 μm at age 30–50 years (Figure 5); and that the hollows increased in diameter from 20–25 μm at age 0–5 years to 35–45 μm at age 30–50 years (Figure 6). These results confirm comparable studies of dry material surveyed under high vacuum by scanning electron microscopy (SEM) (Clarke, 1972).

Articular cartilage thickness
(Armstrong, 1976; Armstrong & Gardner, 1977)

Cartilage surface structure, and its interaction with fluid phases at the surface, determine the lubrication characteristics at a joint and closely influence the 'wear' pattern. The quantity of cartilage, in relation to body mass, mean load, load frequency and joint compliance are among additional physical factors that

69

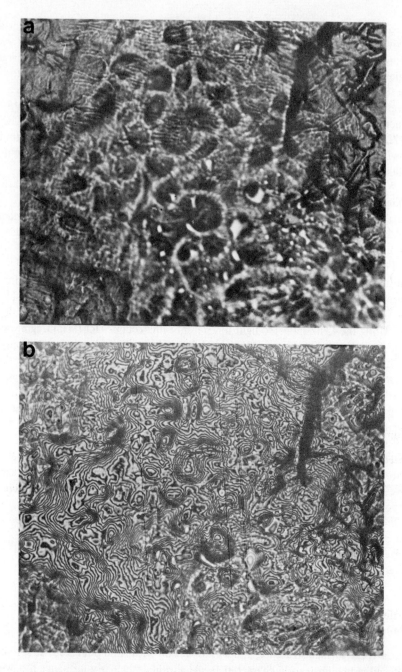

Figure 3 Surface appearances of identical fields of normal articular cartilage of knee
from 20 year old female viewed a) by reflected light microscopy; b) by reflected
light interference microscopy

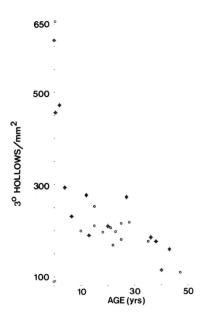

Figure 4   Diagram of tertiary hollow frequency versus age

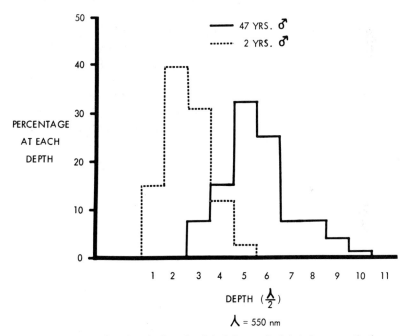

Figure 5   Histogram of tertiary hollow depth in infant and adult in human articular
cartilage

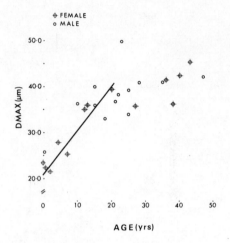

Figure 6   Diagram of tertiary hollow diameter versus age

modulate the response of articular cartilage to the cumulative fatigue factors
that are part of the ageing and of the osteoarthrotic processes. Although we have
not yet been able to measure the cartilage *volume* of femoral heads, we have
successfully measured cartilage *thickness* with much greater precision than has
previously been possible.

Intact femurs were obtained at *postmortem* from subjects aged 10–68 years.
Patients who had a history of chronic renal, metabolic or endocrine disease, of
articular or systemic connective tissue disease, of trauma to the hip joint or
surrounding structures, or of prolonged immobilisation were excluded from the
study, as were those with obesity or overt fibrillation of the femoral head assessed
by India ink painting (Stockwell & Meachim, 1973). Before measurement, each
femur was orientated with respect to the main body planes so that the centre of
the hip joint contact area, approximated by the zenith of the femoral head, was
in the same vertical plane as the tibio-femoral contact area. Accurate orientation

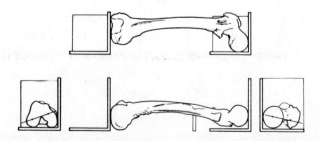

Figure 7   Method used to anatomically orientate the femur

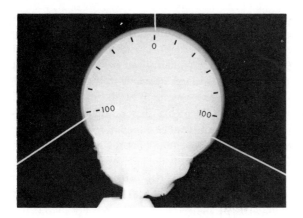

Figure 8   Lateromedial radiograph of a human femoral head

was ensured with a specially designed perspex jig (Figure 7), in which each femur was positioned in a horizontal plane. Contact ink marks on the jig recorded the zenith of the femoral head and the sagittal plane. Femoral head cartilage was displayed in lateromedial radiographs (Figure 8) and its thickness measured to 0.01 mm by means of a Heuer optical projector. The measurement error was ± 0.03mm.

A computer model related cartilage thickness measurements on a linear scale to age, sex, height, weight, femoral head diameter and femoral length. The equations were tested by means of a multiple regression analysis programme.

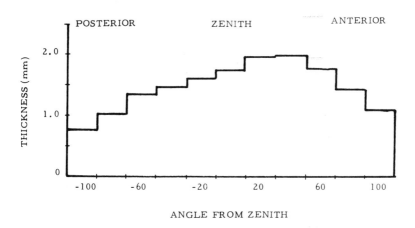

Figure 9 Distribution of the cartilage thickness with angle from the zenith on the
femoral head (degrees)

73

The results of these investigations revealed, first, a characteristic distribution of femoral head cartilage. The thickest zone of cartilage was recognised immediately anterior to the zenith (Figure 9). The distribution of femoral head cartilage was therefore asymmetrical. Asymmetry was least pronounced in immature and young adult femoral head cartilage. Assessments made in several planes showed that there was more cartilage at any point on the anterior hemisphere. In addition, there was more cartilage on the medial than on the lateral surface of the head. Asymmetry was therefore not unique to the lateromedial plane of radiography.

Second, there was little change in thickness with age near the articular margins in adult cartilage. However, towards the anterosuperior surface, cartilage thickness increased up to age 45 years (Figure 10). A maximum was measured in the regions 20° and 40° anterior to the zenith. Thus, the thickest part of the cartilage increased to the greatest extent. The change in thickness was not unique to measurements made in the lateromedial projection plane. Beyond the age of 45 years, the scatter of thickness measurements in this first study precluded valid analysis of material from the 11 oldest subjects.

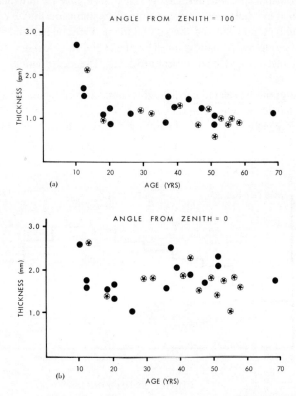

Figure 10   Cartilage thickness variation with age, a) at the cartilage margin; b) at the zenith. (⊕ Males ● Females)

Third, when multiple regression analyses were conducted on those 13 subjects aged 20–45 years, it appeared that cartilage thickness was not significantly influenced by sex, height, weight, femoral head diameter or femoral length. The increase in cartilage thickness at all sites on the anterior half of the femoral head was significantly related only to age, in a simple linear manner. If corrections were performed for specimen dimension, sex and height differences, a significant increase of cartilage thickness with age was also revealed at positions on the femoral head 20° and 40° *posterior* to the zenith.

There is good reason to suggest that the thickening with age of adult femoral head cartilage is one result of the many physiological mechanical loads to which the hip joint is subject during normal life. There is no reason to suppose that trauma causes the rapid onset of increased cartilage thickness other than in a small minority of individuals. It is not easy to draw an analogy with acute animal experiments such as those of McDevitt and Muir (1976), McDevitt et al (1977) and of Muir (1977), in which cartilage injury has been provoked. If, then, a gradual increase in thickness is a response to physiological loading, is this increase a factor predisposing to OA? This is by no means certain. In widely quoted analyses made by the simple but insensitive method of naked eye inspection, Byers et al (1970) described the surface morphology of 375 femoral heads collected at *postmortem*. The collection was biased: all patients were selected for hospital care. Within this limitation, Byers et al found two patterns of crude surface change; 'progressive' (infrequent) and 'limited-progressive' (frequent). 'Progression' was equated with the clinical disease 'osteoarthrosis'. This was assessed, not on the advancement or non-advancement of individual cases but by extrapolation from the survey at single points in time in the 375 cases.

Morphologically, 'progressive lesions' were present on the superior surface of only 16 of the 375 femoral heads. Nevertheless in 15 of these 16 examples, these changes were anterosuperior. It appears then, that although the antero-superior femoral head cartilage thickens with age, this zone becomes the site of 'progressive' change ('disease') in only a minority of persons.

Articular cartilage compliance
(Armstrong, 1977; Armstrong et al, 1977a, b)

In the walking cycle, the maximum forces imposed on a hip joint range from 4.9 x body weight during slow movement to 7.6 x body weight during fast movement. In each walking cycle, these peaks are imposed twice, at the 'heel-strike' and 'toe-off' positions. The physical changes in cartilage structure in response to these forces are of the greatest interest.

The considerable published evidence on the deformability of articular cartilage is derived from tests with methods that lead to very large strains. Indeed in *tension* tests, strains as large as 100 per cent have been observed (Woo et al, 1976). The superior surface of the human femoral head is covered by a band of cartilage stiffer than that covering the remainder of the joint (Kempson et al, 1971). In the stiff area the short-term Young's modulus is normally in the range 6–10 MN m^{-2}. In indentation tests of femoral heads from patients aged 26–83 years, no change in the short-term Young's modulus for cartilage was found with advancing age (Armstrong, 1977). These observations shed no light on the distribution of stress patterns within the hip joint, and in particular, fail to elucidate integrated cartilage change of a form that is likely to occur during life. There seemed a clear case for more sophisticated surveys, testing the whole hip joint, making exact measurements of changes in cartilage contours, and employing loading forces comparable to those known to obtain in vivo.

For this purpose a method was devised that allowed changes in cartilage contours in the whole joint to be measured under conditions simulating those encountered during life. This procedure offered an alternative to the technically difficult task of recording the distribution of pressure within the loaded joint bearing surfaces.

An hydraulic power pack conveyed pressurised oil to a loading rig in which a servo-controlled hydraulic piston applied loads to mounted specimens. The total displacement of the specimen was measured by a transducer incorporated in the specimen mounting. X-rays were taken of the loaded and unloaded joints. The applied load, the specimen displacement and the X-ray exposure time were recorded.

Twenty-eight specimens from subjects aged 26–83 years were collected, stored temporarily at -20° and tested at a room temperature. To permit comparisons of different X-rays, pins were fixed as reference points on the femoral head circumference. Tests were made in a standard orientation relative to the peak force at the toe-off position in the walking cycle. Cartilage deformation could be measured radiographically by introducing Dionosil Oily with phosphotringstic acid into the hip joint, allowing the cartilage interface to be located exactly. X-rays taken under these conditions before and after loading were measured by an electronic signal processing unit and monitor, which enabled cartilage thickness at defined sites around the circumference to be measured to within 1%.

The experimental evidence that the Young's modulus E for the cartilage examined did not vary suggested that the magnitude of cartilage deformations in the whole joint would be similar at all ages. This was not so. Further, the average strain was found to be much less than that calculated from the values for Young's modulus. The average strain was expected to be ca. 15%. However, this was found to be a maximum value for the most compliant cartilage.

Cartilage compliance increases with age in a highly significant manner (Figure 11). There was no relation between compliance and sex, weight, height, femoral head diameter, Young's modulus for cartilage and maximum femoral head cartilage thickness even after the variation with age had been removed by multiple regression analysis. During longer loading periods of up to 40 minutes, a general trend towards increasing deformation with time was also observed. There was no

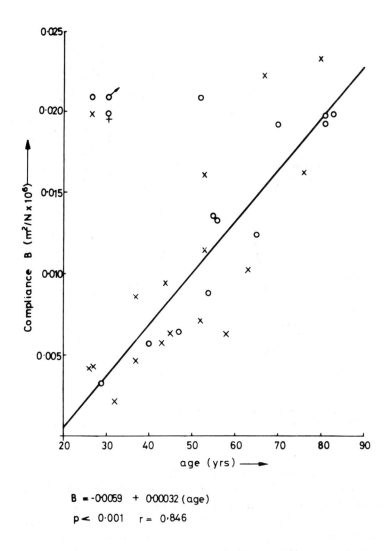

$$B = -0.0059 + 0.00032 \, (age)$$

$$p < 0.001 \qquad r = 0.846$$

Figure 11 Relationship of cartilage compliance with age in the femoral head

correlation of the measured value of compliance (total deformation per *unit* load) with the applied load or the average pressure applied.

The data (Figure 12) demonstrate that young cartilage is very difficult to compress: a large load is required to overcome the normal incongruity of the hip joint, allowing complete contact between the femoral head and the acetabulum. Although, in old hip joints the surfaces are still incongruent, relatively small loads only are required to bring the surfaces into complete contact.

These results suggest mechanical and/or biochemical changes in femoral head

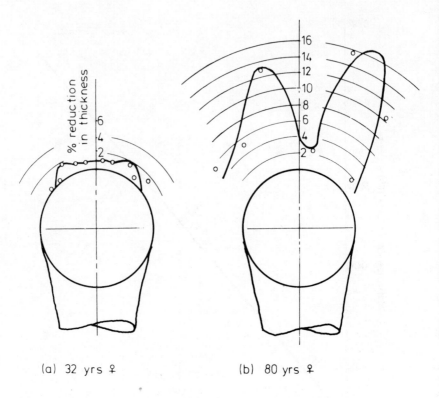

(a) 32 yrs ♀   (b) 80 yrs ♀

Figure 12   Distribution of the deformation of femoral head cartilage for a load of five times body weight. Lateromedial projection. Left — female, 32 years; right — female, 80 years.

articular cartilage microstructure with age. They offer guidance towards the identification of the mode of failure of cartilage as a bearing material. The fatigue failure of cartilage has been attributed to collagen microfractures (Freeman, 1975; Weightman, 1976). The recent work of Brandt and Palmoski (1976) and of McDevitt et al (1977) suggests that with increasing age, or with the onset of cartilage failure in osteoarthrosis, the proteoglycan aggregates are much reduced in size; the proportion of proteoglycan in monomer forms is increased; and the proportion of proteoglycan tightly bound to collagen is much decreased. This evidence supports the concept that either collagen defects, or proteoglycan changes, or a disturbance of the collagen/proteoglycan interface determines the mechanical failure of cartilage. If the alterations demonstrated by Brandt and Palmoski (1976) can be shown to be age-related, then the cumulative deficiencies of the collagen/ proteoglycan interface can reasonably be suggested as the explanation for the increasing compliance and diminishing load-bearing efficiency that characterises ageing human femoral head articular cartilage.

Articular cartilage composition
(Elliott, 1976; Elliott & Gardner 1975, 1977a, 1977b).

The evidence presented in the previous sections leads to the hypothesis that the failure of articular cartilage as a load-bearing material is attributable to the cumulative modification of individual molecular components or of their composite form. Normal femoral condylar cartilage contains about 70% water. Of the solid

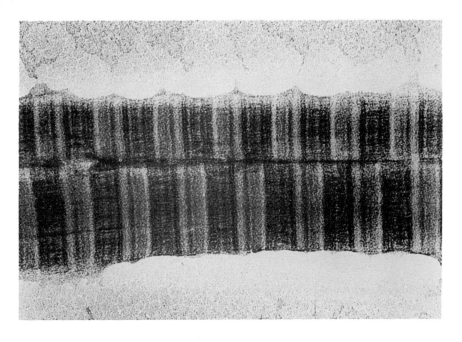

Figure 13 Electron micrograph of Type II collagen isolated from human articular cartilage (x 225,000)

components, 48–62% is type II collagen, (Figure 13), the remainder being glyco-saminoglycan (9–23%) arranged upon core proteins, glycoproteins, inorganic salts (1%) and unidentified molecules (up to 30% of the dry weight) (Kempson et al, 1970).

That mechanical failure of articular cartilage is attributable to a failure of collagen fibre organisation has been discussed. The possibility of failure of the proteoglycans (Figure 14) or of their aggregates has emerged (Kempson et al, 1968, 1971; Brandt & Palmoski, 1976). The theory that mechanical fatigue failure of articular cartilage is a disorder of the proteoglycan – collagen interaction has also to be considered.

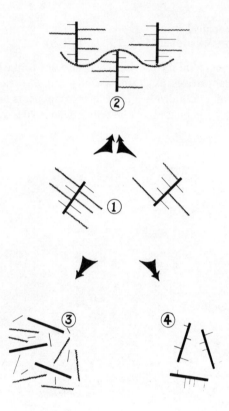

Figure 14   A diagrammatic outline of articular cartilage proteoglycans based on electron microscopy and enzyme assay evidence.

1.   The proteoglycan monomer is formed from a polypeptide core and carbohydrate side chains (glycosaminoglycans). In adult cartilage the proteoglycan monomer side chains are chondroitin sulphate and keratan sulphate.

2.   In vivo and under controlled test-tube conditions the proteoglycan monomers can, in the presence of hyaluronic acid and link protein(s), form a macromolecular aggregate. The peptide core of the monomers is attached to the hyaluronic acid molecule in the presence of the link protein(s).

3.   Proteoglycans can be rapidly taken apart by the action of cold dilute alkali. The alkali reacts with the serine residues to release the glycosaminoglycans from the peptide core.

4.   Alternatively, the glycosaminoglycan side chains can be selectively removed using cleavage enzymes. Chondroitin sulphate, for example, can be removed specifically by chondroitin ABC lyase (E.C.4.2.2.4.).

The proteoglycan components represented in this figure are not to scale. From electron microscopy examination the following mean values have been obtained.

Length of hyaluronate backbone	4,200 nm
peptide core	300 nm
chondroitin sulphate chain	40 nm
keratan sulphate chain	15 nm

80

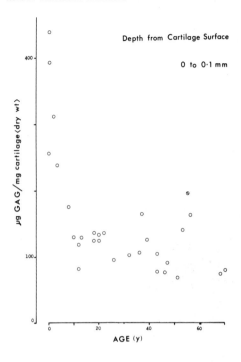

Figure 15   The change with age in the total glycosaminoglycan content of human
femoral cartilage

Searching for evidence to support or refute these views, Elliott (1976) investigated the lateral femoral condylar cartilage of 60 samples of 30 normal human
subjects aged 0–70 years. The glycosaminoglycan (GAG) composition of the
specimens was examined in two 100 μm thick zones, the first from the surface
downwards, the second at a depth of 900–1000 μm from the surface.

At birth *total* GAG content (Figure 15) accounted for 50% of the dry weight
of the superficial and intermediate zones of cartilage. This value rapidly declined
to 10–20% at age 10 years. This figure was maintained throughout normal life,
with a characteristic increase in scatter recognisable after the age of 40 years.
When these 100 μm thick samples are compared, the GAG concentrations for
the deeper zone differ little from those for the superficial (Elliott & Gardner,
1977a, b). This does not exclude the likelihood, deduced from histochemical
observations, that the most superficial cartilage zone, down to 20 μm from the
surface, contains relatively little GAG; an observation concealed when sampling
tangential slices as large as 100 μm.

81

Chondroitin sulphate accounts for almost all the GAG found in articular cartilage at birth: there is little change in this relative concentration for the first 20 years i.e. until growth ceases, when chondroitin sulphate comes to represent about 85% of total cartilage GAG. This value decreases little during the remainder of life in normal individuals. It is important to note that there is much more variation in the proportion of GAG represented by chondroitin sulphate in the superficial than in the deep zone sampled; an observation that supports the concept of an age-related progressive alteration in that part of the cartilage that first displays the changes of osteoarthrosis.

The keratan sulphate content of the cartilage increases slowly during the growth period to reach about 15% of the total cartilage GAG at age 20 years. In the deeper cartilage little further change occurs during the remainder of adult life. There is a much greater variation in values for the superficial, 100 μm zone, where keratan sulphate can reach higher relative proportions (up to 20–30%) compared to deep zone cartilage.

The presence of small quantities of hyaluronic acid (HA) in human articular cartilage has attracted rapidly increasing attention in recent years (Elliott & Gardner, 1975). In measurements made by Elliott (1976) on the samples at 0–100 μm and at 900–1000 μm deep to the surface, it appears first that detectable amounts of HA are not present at birth; second that HA exceeds 1% of total cartilage GAG only after skeletal growth creases; and third, that there is a continual linear increase in relative HA concentration, reaching 6% of the GAG by age 60 years. Greater concentrations of HA are present in deep zone (900–1000 μm) cartilage than in superficial, and the relationship to age is identical for the HA of both zones.

These age changes in articular cartilage glycosaminoglycans reveal that the proteoglycans are neither stable nor of uniform composition. Because of the importance of PG in retaining water and for controlling the movement of metabolites into and out of the cartilage, it is possible that these unique molecules can explain how articular cartilage withstands weight-bearing and frictional stresses encountered throughout life.

Conclusions

Our recent investigations show that in human femoral head or femoral condylar articular cartilage there are changes with age in:
   — the depth and diameter of the surface tertiary hollows of the lateral condyle;
   — the thickness of the thickest zones of femoral head cartilage;
   — the deformability (compliance) of femoral head cartilage in response to physiological loads:
   — the content of the condylar cartilage GAG, in particular the HA, of both superficial and deep condylar cartilage.

These observations greatly extend those in the literature. They begin to define a pattern that can logically relate age to mechanical failure.

References

Armstrong CG (1976) *Clinical Science and Molecular Medicine, 50,* 1

Armstrong CG (1977) *Ph.D. Thesis,* the Queen's University of Belfast

Armstrong CG, Bahrani AS and Gardner DL (1977a) *Lancet, I,* 1103

Armstrong CG, Bahrani AS and Gardner DL (1977b) *Proceedings of American Society of Mechanical Engineers Symposium on Biomechanics.* In press

Armstrong CG and Gardner DL (1977) *Annals of the Rheumatic Diseases, 36,* 407

Brandt KD and Palmoski M (1976) *Arthritis and Rheumatism, 19,* 209

Byers PD, Contemponi CA and Farkas TA (1970) *Annals of the Rheumatic Diseases, 29,*15

Clarke IC (1972) *Ph.D. Thesis,* The University of Strathclyde

Davies DV (1969) In *Textbook of the Rheumatic Diseases.* Ed. WSC Copeman, 4th edition, Livingstone, Edinburgh, p.25

Dowson D, Longfield MD, Walker PS and Wright V (1968) *Proceedings of the Institution of Mechanical Engineers, 181, 3J,* 16

Elliott RJ (1976) *Ph.D. Thesis,* The Queen's University of Belfast

Elliott RJ and Gardner DL (1975) *10th Meeting of the Federation of European Biochemical Societies (FEBS), Paris, Abstract 920.* Published by La Societe de Chimie Biologique, Paris

Elliott RJ and Gardner DL (1977a) *Biochimica et Biophysica Acta, 498,* 349

Elliott RJ and Gardner DL (1977b) *Analytical Biochemistry.* In press

Freeman MAR (1975) *Acta Orthopaedica Scandinavica, 46,* 323

Gardner DL (1972a) In *8th Symposium on Advanced Medicine.* Ed. G Neale. Pitman Medical, London. P.353

Gardner DL (1972b) *Annals of the Rheumatic Diseases, 31,* 235

Gardner DL and Longmore RB (1974) In *Normal and Osteoarthrotic Articular Cartilage.* Eds. SY Ali, MW Elves and DH Leaback, Institute of Orthopaedics, London. P. 141

Gardner DL and Woodward DH (1968) *Lancet 2,* 1246

Glynn LE (1977) *Lancet, I,* 574

Inoue H, Kodama T and Fujita T (1969) *Archivum Histologicum Japonicum, 30,* 425

Kempson GE (1973) In *Adult Articular Cartilage.* Ed. MAR Freeman, Pitman Medical, London

Kempson GE, Freeman MAR and Swanson SAV (1968) *Nature 220,* 1127

Kempson GE, Freeman MAR and Swanson SAV (1971) *Journal of Biomechanics, 4,* 239

Kempson GE, Muir H, Swanson SAV and Freeman MAR (1970) *Biochimica et Biophysica Acta, 215,* 70

Kirkpatrick CJ and Gardner DL (1977) *Experientia, 34,* 504

Longmore RB (1976) *Ph.D. Thesis,* The Queen's University of Belfast

Longmore RB, and Gardner DL (1975) *Annals of the Rheumatic Diseases, 34,* 26

Longmore RB and Gardner DL (1977) *Journal of Microscopy*

McCall JG (1968) *M.Sc. Thesis,* The University of Strathclyde

McDevitt C and Muir H (1976) *Journal of Bone and Joint Surgery, 58–B,* 94

McDevitt C, Gilbertson E and Muir H (1977) *Journal of Bone and Joint Surgery, 59–B*

Meachim G (1971) *Annals of the Rheumatic Diseases, 30,* 43

Mow VC, Lai WM, Eisenfield J and Redler I (1974) *Journal of Biomechanics, 7,* 457

Muir H (1977) *Annals of the Rheumatic Diseases, 36,* 199

Radin EL (1974) In *The Hip, Proceedings of the Second Open Scientific Meeting of the Hip Society.* Ed. WH Harris, C V Mosby Company, St Louis

Simon WH, Friedenberg S and Richardson S (1973) *Journal of Bone and Joint Surgery, 55–A,* 1614

Sokoloff L (1968) *Federation Proceedings, 25,* 1089

Stockwell RA and Meachim G (1973) In *Adult Articular Cartilage.* Ed. MAR Freeman, Pitman Medical, London

Unsworth A, Dowson D and Wright V (1975) *Annals of the Rheumatic Diseases, 34,* 277

Weightman B (1976) *Journal of Biomechanics, 9,* 193

Woo SL-Y, Akeson WH and Jemmott GF (1976) *Journal of Biomechanics, 9,* 785

8

OSTEOARTHROSIS AS A FINAL COMMON PATHWAY

Eric L Radin, Igor L Paul, Robert M Rose

Introduction

We basically hold with the view that osteoarthrosis (we prefer this term over 'degenerative joint disease' for reasons we have outlined in a previous publication (Radin et al, 1976)) is the result of an imbalance between the stress applied to the joint and its ability to tolerate that stress. Osteoarthrosis therefore must be viewed as a relationship between mechanical and biological factors.

Anyone who attempts to suggest that osteoarthrosis is caused by a single factor, be it congenital, developmental, vascular or traumatic is a fanatic and should be treated as such. There is no question that these factors can play an aetiological role but those who contend that such factors are always present and that primary osteoarthrosis is a myth are wrong. Such conclusions are based on retrospective studies of hip x-rays of patients who developed severe coxarthrosis (Murray, 1965). First of all the hip joint is the most prone in the body to develop congenital, developmental and vascular problems, and secondly, it is extremely difficult to determine in retrospect which changes in anatomy are from secondary remodelling and which are actually primary. A large proportion of osteoarthrosis occurs without obvious pre-existing cause.

What then can cause articular cartilage to deteriorate. Cartilage can be destroyed by proteolytic and glycolytic enzymes which can be produced by synovial inflammation. However, such enzyme producing inflammation appears to be secondary to cartilage damage, and although a contributing cause of cartilage wear enzymatic activity would not appear to be the initiating cause (Bollet, 1969). Disuse can result in articular cartilage deterioration. The habitually non-loaded articular cartilage, usually peripheral in a joint, commonly fibrillates (Harrison et al, 1953), but this fibrillation tends not to be progressive; that is this cartilage tends not to wear away. Cartilage in the habitually loaded areas of joints, once fibrillated, tends to be progressively worn (Foss & Byers, 1972).

Finally, while on the subject of dismissing 'old rheumatologists' tales' on the aetiology of osteoarthrosis we should mention ageing. Although it is comfortable to think of joints as just 'wearing out from old age', they don't (Sokoloff, 1969). There is an increasing incidence of osteoarthrosis with ageing, but the evidence so far is most consistant with the hypothesis that mechanical factors are related to the progressive destruction of articular cartilage. This suggests that stress history, or accumulated stress, is what provides the correlation between age and osteoarthrosis (Radin, 1976).

Car accidents and skiing injuries normally do not cause osteoarthrosis, rather it is the stress generated by the activities of daily living and the ability of the tissues to withstand these stresses. Therefore we can have osteoarthrosis in instances where the dynamic force in the joint is increased because of altered anatomy or situations where the tissue resistance to stress is lowered (Pauwels, 1965). The latter, lowered tissue resistance to stress, can involve either the bony or cartilagenous structures of the joint itself, or the other musculo-skeletal shock absorbers that normally protect joints from expected stresses.

Factors Tending to Increase the Stress on Cartilage

If stress history is a significant variable in the cause of cartilage degeneration in osteoarthrosis, what is the nature and quantity of such stress? First let us discuss its quantity. High peak amplitude stress causes fracture of bone. Unless the fracture goes into the joint and results in an incongruity or chondral injury, or the fracture heals with angulation in such a way that the normal alignment of the joint is disturbed, no late osteoarthrosis occurs.

1.   *Instances Where the Stress is Increased*
a.   Congenital or Development Abnormalities of the Joint.
This is most easily appreciated in the knee. Varus or valgus deformities at the knee will eventually lead to osteoarthrosis of the compartment of the knee that is subject to its unfair share of load. The hip joint is probably subject to more congenital and developmental abnormality than any other joint in the body and such deformities unquestionably contribute to many cases of coxarthrosis.

Whatever the cause, a loss of cartilage contact area will increase the force per unit area on the remaining contact area. If high enough such a concentration of stress on the articular cartilage may make it difficult for the chondrocytes to continue to function properly and inactivate whatever other factors in the extracellular matrix cause proper aggregation and orientation of the matrix macromolecules. The cells keep trying, at least while they are still around (Mankin & Lipiello, 1970), but the increased mechanical stress makes it impossible for them to succeed. Even in cases where fibrocartilagenous healing does occur, the junction between such tissue and normal cartilage is a point of concentration and breakdown eventually occurs (Rosenberg, personal communication). One is much

85

better off for a long-term bearing surface with complete fibrocartilage than fibro-cartilagenous areas interspersed with normal articular cartilage (Radin et al, 1975). Two unlike materials concentrate shear and pull apart at their junction.

b. Traumatic Lesions of Joints
Significant osteochondral injuries, post-traumatic incongruities or mal-alignments will lead to joint degeneration. Here again there is a lack of available articular bearing surface. The remainder of the surface has to take a greater share of the load. The stress is concentrated.

2.   *Instances Where the Stress is Normal but the Tissue Resistance to Stress is Lowered*   Theoretically there should be instances where the tissue tolerance has been lowered and the tissues are unable to handle usual levels of stress. As far as the subchondral bone is concerned, osteopenia and osteoporosis both increase the brittleness of bone, making it a far better shock absorber than normal bone. Fracture of bone is a very elegant shock absorbing mechanism and protects the cartilage from deterioration (Byers et al, 1970). Rickets, Paget's Disease, Acro-megly, and Gaucher's Disease are examples of metabolic or endocrine abnormalities that can lead to joint incongruity.

Cartilage can deteriorate. Infection and certain metabolic processes, e.g.chon-drocalcinosis which affect cartilage can significantly alter the tissues ability to handle normal stress. Ochronosis is an example of a disease which can lower the mechanical resistance of the cartilage probably by stiffening it and is a cause of obvious secondary osteoarthrosis.

3.   *Inadequate Shock Absorption*   The major protective mechanism acting to spare articular cartilage from peak dynamic loading appears to be joint motion with resultant lengthening of muscles under tension (Jones & Watt, 1971). This is all reflexly controlled and happens naturally. As long as we have time for the reflexes to get ready, which is in humans about 75 milliseconds, physiologic loading can be damped sufficiently so that there will be no damage to the articular cartilage.

Deformation of bone and soft tissue also contribute (Radin & Paul, 1970). Soft tissues and bone attenuate peak forces most effectively at higher frequency ranges and these components compliment the stretching of muscle under tension, which is more effective at lower frequency ranges. Soft tissues contribute to peak force attenuation over the entire physiologic frequency spectrum (Paul, I L et al, unpublished observations).

The Nature of the Destructive Stress on Articular Cartilage

It is difficult, from surveying the clinical situations which can cause cartilage destruction, to determine what sort of stress need be involved in order for carti-lage to wear. We know that fibrillation alone is not enough (Meachim, 1963), that constant rubbing has no deleterious effect (Radin & Paul, 1971), and that repetitive longitudinal loading will not damage cartilage (Radin et al, 1976a). If we study the physiologically reasonable mechanical models by which joints can be experimentally damaged, a pattern emerges.

The experimental methods are: subluxation (Hulth et al, 1970), removal of all the cartilage (Kettunen, 1958), creation of a joint incongruity or abnormal pressure distribution (Ito et al, 1968: Moskowitz et al, 1973), creation of a stiffness gradient in the subchondral bone (Radin et al, 1976b), and over-riding the natural shock-absorbing mechanisms (Simon et al, 1972).

1.   *Sublux the Joint*   Subluxation causes high *shear* stresses within the cartilage as it is caught between the incongruous bony outlines as the joint slides in and out of its normal orientation.

2.   *Remove Significant Amounts of Loadbearing Cartilage*   Under these circumstances the opposing cartilage will rub against bone which is somewhat irregular and is only one tenth as deformable as the cartilage which it now replaces. This will have an abrasive effect on the remaining articular cartilage, create significant *shear* stress in it, and cause it to deteriorate.

3.   *Create a Joint Incongruity or Abnormal Pressure Distribution Within a Joint*   The absence of a condyle, a torn meniscus or mal-fitting surfaces will either cause a decrease in contact area or an irregular distribution of the stress within the joint. The stress on some regions of the cartilage is therefore increased. Because of the irregularity of the stress distribution within the joint under these circumstances the cartilage in some areas will be deformed more than others and will be subjected to *shear* stress.

4.   *Create a Stiffness Gradient in the Underlying Subchondral Bone*   As cartilage is compressed, that over relatively stiff bone will be deformed more than cartilage over relatively more deformable bone. This will create a *shear* stress in the cartilage just overlying the area of stiffness gradient in the bone.

The amount of shear stress created will depend upon the degree of the stiffness gradient in the bone. A significant stiffness gradient will create considerable shear in the cartilage.

5.   *Over-ride the Natural Shock Absorbing Mechanisms During Physiological Loading*   The activities of daily living create impulsive loads on oscillating joints. If one inhibits joint motion distal to the loaded joint, by a splint or arthrodesis, then the natural major shock absorbing mechanism, joint motion causing a pull on tensed muscle, cannot function. The full force of the impulsive load is felt. If done repetitively and always in the same orientation of the joint excessive microfracture of the cancellous bone will occur creating an area of stiffened underlying bone. *Shear* stresses in the cartilage will result.

Clearly what all these models have in common is the creation of shear stress within the cartilage, which normally sees little because of the low frictional resistances at its surface (Radin, 1968) and the organisation of its attachment to calcified cartilage (Redler et al, 1975). In vitro cartilage can easily be sheared away with such stress applied on a repetative basis (Radin & Paul, 1971).

Present Viewpoint

Mechanical factors are involved in progressive cartilage wear. Cartilage fibrillation can be non-progressive. For fibrillation to become progressive it must be in a weightbearing area. But not all weightbearing cartilage fibrillation is progressive (Abernethy et al, 1976), and weightbearing alone will not cause cartilage destruction. The culprit would appear to be the level of shear stress in the cartilage. Unless there is some abnormality, significant shear stresses are not created by oscillating a joint. What is needed to create shear stress is a stiffness gradient in the cartilage or in its underlying bone. This can be caused by a variety of factors: loss of significant cartilage substance, a torn meniscus, incongruity, subluxation, or healing of an excessive number of microfractures in the underlying bone. The latter can result from quite subtle failures of shock absorption and can result from trivial trauma (Radin et al, 1976a). Cartilage is destroyed by shear stress. Osteoarthrosis represents the common final pathway of a variety of mechanisms all of which involve an imbalance between the stress applied to joints and the normal ability of the various tissues of the limbs to attenuate this stress so that the cartilage can tolerate it.

Although it was formally thought that lowered cartilage tolerance to such stress was the commonest cause of osteoarthrosis, except in certain well defined systemic metabolic abnormalities, even damaged cartilage can survive if the stress level is tolerable. The most likely culprit in idiopathic osteoarthrosis is the subchondral bone. Stiffened subchondral bone can cause a dramatic increase in the wear rate of articular cartilage in vitro (Radin et al, 1976b), and the earliest metabolic and chemical changes in articular cartilage, in vivo, are associated with a significant stiffening of the subchondral bone (Radin et al, 1977). Increased stiffening of underlying subchondral bone is probably the most likely agent responsible for the progressive wear of fibrillated cartilage in primary osteoarthrosis, although other factors may be involved.

Acknowledgment

This work was supported by the National Institute of Arthritis, Metabolic and Digestive Diseases.

References

Abernethy,PJ, Townsend,PR, Rose,RM, and Radin,EL (1976) *Proceedings of the American Rheumatism Association, Miami Beach.* Page 42

Bollet, AJ, (1969) *Arthritis and Rheumatism, 12,* 152

Byers, PD, Contepomi, CA, and Farkas, TA, (1970) *Annals of Rheumatic Diseases, 29,* 15

Foss, MVL, and Byers, PD, (1972) *Annals of Rheumatic Diseases, 31,* 259

Harrison, MHM, Schajowicz, F, and Trueta, J, (1953) *Journal of Bone and Joint Surgery, 35B,* 598

Hulth, A, Lindberg, L, and Telhag, H (1970) *Acta Orthopaedica Scandinavica, 41,* 522

Ito, T, Kokosaki, M, and Nakamasu, M (1968) *Acta Orthopaedica Scandinavica, 39,* 518

Jones, GM, and Watt, DGD (1971) *Journal of Physiology, 219,* 729

Kettunen, KO (1958) *Acta Orthopaedica Scandinavica Supplement 29*

Mankin, HJ, and Lipiello, L (1970) *Journal of Bone and Joint Surgery, 52A,* 424

Meachim, G (1963) *Journal of Bone and Joint Surgery, 45B,* 150

Moskowitz, RW, Davis, WD, Sammarco, J, Martens, M, Baker, J, Mayor, M, Burstein, AH and Frankel, VH (1973) *Arthritis and Rheumatism, 16,* 397

Murray, RO (1965) *British Journal of Radiology, 38,* 810

Pauwels, F (1965) *Gesammelte Abhandlungen zur functionellen Anatomie des Bewegungsapparates.* Springer-Verlag, Berlin

Radin, EL (1968) *Arthritis and Rheumatism, 11,* 693

Radin, EL (1976) *Bulletin on the Rheumatic Diseases, 26,* 862

Radin, EL, Ehrlich, MG, Chernack, RS, Paul, IL, and Rose, RM (1977) *Proceedings Orthopaedic Research Society, Las Vegas.* Page 74

Radin, EL, Ehrlich, MM, Weiss, CA, and Parker, GH (1976) *Recent Advances in Rheumatology.* (Ed) W Watson Buchanan and W Carson Dick. Churchill-Livingstone, London. Page 1

Radin, EL, Maquet, P, and Parker, H (1975) *Clinical Orthopaedics, 112,* 221

Radin, EL, Paul, IL, Rose, RM, and Simon, SR (1976a) *American Academy of Orthopaedic Surgeons Symposium on Osteoarthrosis.* CV Mosby, St Louis. Page 34

Radin, EL, Myttas, NJ, Swann, DA, and Paul, IL (1976b) *Proceedings American Rheumatism Association, Miami Beach.* Page 49

Radin, EL, and Paul, IL (1971) *Arthritis and Rheumatism, 14,* 356

Redler, I, Zimny, ML, Mansell, J, and Mow, VC (1975) *Clinical Orthopaedics, 112,* 357

Simon, SR, Radin, EL, and Paul, IL (1972) *Journal of Biomechanics, 5,* 267

Sokoloff, L (1969) *The Biology of Degenerative Joint Disease.* University of Chicago Press

9

THE PATHOGENESIS OF IDIOPATHIC ('PRIMARY') OSTEOARTHROSIS: AN HYPOTHESIS

M A R Freeman

In this chapter the hypothesis is advanced that osteoarthrosis (OA) is the non-specific end result of a number of pathological processes which have in common the fact that they destroy articular cartilage. As such OA could be viewed as 'joint failure', analogous to heart failure. At an early stage in the evolution of idiopathic osteoarthrosis the articular cartilage develops surface defects (i.e. fibrillation). Although fibrillation always precedes frank osteoarthrosis and its incidence, like that of idiopathic OA, rises with advancing age, it appears that fibrillation does not always progress to osteoarthrosis. It is now suggested that the fatigue strength of the fibre network in cartilage falls with advancing age, thus accounting for the increased incidence of fibrillation and idiopathic OA in the elderly.

That the mechanical properties of the fibre network in cartilage deteriorate with advancing age may be demonstrated by static tensile tests (Kempson, 1975) or, more dramatically, by tensile fatigue tests (Weightman, 1976). The following lines of argument suggest that this deterioration in the mechanical properties of the network is responsible for fibrillation and eventually for OA.

(1) A loss of tensile strength (static and fatigue) is so far the only age-related abnormality to be demonstrated in intact articular cartilage.

Since fibrillation is also age-related, this suggests, but does not prove, that the two are causally connected and, since a loss of tensile strength (static and fatigue) can be demonstrated in *intact* cartilage, it also suggests that fibre network 'deterioration', revealed by a loss of tensile strength, precedes fibrillation.

(2) Fibrillation consists morphologically of matrix fragmentation, and this must imply the presence of multiple ruptures in the fibre network. Thus any abnormality which weakens the fibre network might be reasonably considered as a possible precursor of fibrillation.

(3) Since overt fibrillation is known to spread tangentially over the articular surface, it is reasonable to seek its precursor in areas of intact cartilage adjacent

to areas of fibrillation. The tensile fatigue properties of such cartilage have not yet been examined, but its static tensile strength and stiffness are variably diminished (Kempson, unpublished observations). These abnormalities demonstrate an abnormality of the fibre network.

(4) The Indian ink stained surface of cartilage which has been subjected to a cyclical compressive load in vitro may display appearances similar to the *en face* appearances of some forms of 'minimal' fibrillation (Weightman et al, 1973).

(5) The total uncalcified thickness of cartilage showing histological evidence of surface fraying appears to be slightly greater than that of cartilage on which the surface is histologically intact (Meachim, 1971) and its water content is increased (Venn & Maroudas 1977; Maroudas & Venn unpublished observations) i.e. it is swollen or oedematous. Since the collagen fibre network has a low elasticity, cartilage can not swell significantly whilst this network is intact. Thus the swelling of the tissue would imply a fibre network abnormality (i.e. increased distensibility attributable to fragmentation). In keeping with this interpretation, results from transmission electron microscopy (Meachim & Roy, 1969; Ficat, 1975) indicate that, in man, fibrillation may be preceded by an ultrastructural state in which there is abnormally wide separation, fragmentation and disorientation of the collagen fibres of the superficial cartilage layer. It is of interest that Ficat (1975) has observed a similar ultrastructural 'oedema' in the softened cartilage on the patella in Chondromalacia Patellae.

(6) In a canine experimental model of osteoarthrosis, the first detectable abnormality seen before fibrillation is demonstrable by Indian ink staining of the surface, is once again an increase in the thickness and water content of the cartilage, accompanied by a qualitative change in proteoglycan synthesis (McDevitt et al, 1977). The increased hydration of the tissue again implies increased distensibility of, and, hence mechanical changes in, the fibre network. As in man wide separation and apparent fragmentation of the collagen fibres can be seen with the electron microscope.

(7) If age-related fibrillation in man is the result of a mechanical deterioration in the collagen network of hyaline articular cartilage, a phenomenon similar to fibrillation might also be expected to occur in other collagenous tissues subjected to a similar mechanical environment. A recent study of the fibrocartilaginous menisci of the human knee (Meachim, unpublished observations) has shown that these structures do in fact undergo an age-related process of fraying and splitting, several features of which are similar to those seen in fibrillation of hyaline articular cartilage.

It is interesting to speculate as to the cause of the age-related mechanical abnormalities in the fibre network in cartilage. It is known that the fibre of which this network is composed is collagen and that collagen turnover occurs very slowly if at all in human adult articular cartilage (Libby et al, 1964; Maroudas unpublished observations). Collagenase is thought to be absent from normal cartilage, although Cathepsin B, which is present, does degrade collagen to a slight extent. For these reasons it seems unlikely that a metabolically induced abnormality in the collagen fibres themselves is responsible for weakening the network. On the other hand, the very inertness of collagen suggests the possibility of its being degraded mechanically rather than chemically, since over the course of a lifetime each fibre will experience a very large number of load cycles whilst the network is now known to be fatigue-prone (Weightman, 1976). Although progressive fatigue failure of the collagen fibres *themselves* may play a part in the age-related weakening of the fibre network, it cannot however be the main factor responsible, since the shortening of the fatigue life in aged cartilage as compared with that in youth is too great to be accounted for by the number of load cycles borne by the fibres in the intervening years (Weightman, 1976). Thus it seems possible, even likely, that the fundamental event in fatigue failure of the fibre network does not concern the individual collagen fibres as such, but instead concerns the 'links' between them.

Virtually nothing is known of the way in which individual fibres are linked to produce a network capable of resisting tension: possibly the fibres are simply interlocked physically, or possibly some other constituent of the matrix functions as a 'glue'. If the latter proves to be the case, abnormalities in the 'bonding' constituent, which might in quantitative terms be an insignificant component of the matrix, could be responsible for the loss of network strength, and might have a metabolic basis.

Summary

Reference is made to studies already in the literature which demonstrate that the fibre network in cartilage is fatigue-prone and that its tensile fatigue strength, falls with advancing age.

Fibrillation of cartilage precedes the development of idiopathic OA, although it does not always progress to OA. A number of observations, reviewed in this paper, suggest that fibrillation, and hence OA, is the macroscopic manifestation of fatigue failure in the fibre network.

The speculation is advanced that the loss of fatigue-strength in the fibre network is probably due mainly to disruption of the bonds between collagen fibres rather than to fragmentation of the fibres themselves.

References

Ficat P (1975) *Annals of the Rheumatic Diseases, 34,* supplement 2, 125
Kempson GE (1975) *Annals of the Rheumatic Diseases, 34,* supplement 2, 111
Libby WF, Berger R, Mead JF, Alexander GV and Ross JF (1964) *Science, 146,* 1170
McDevitt C, Gilbertson E and Muir H (1977) *Journal of Bone and Joint Surgery, 59B,* 24
Meachim G (1971) *Journal of Pathology, 107,* 199
Venn M and Maroudas A (1977) *Annals of the Rheumatic Diseases, 36,* 121
Weightman B (1976) *Journal of Biomechanics, 9,* 193
Weightman B, Freeman MAR and Swanson SAV (1973) *Nature, 224,* 303

10

OSTEOARTHRITIS: SPECULATIONS ON SOME BIOCHEMICAL FACTORS OF POSSIBLE AETIOLOGICAL NATURE INCLUDING CARTILAGE MINERALISATION

D S Howell

Most biochemical pathways uncovered in cartilage during the last two decades describe tissue responses in osteoarthritis to aetiological factors of an extremely complex nature. Those biochemical processes on which the most emphasis has been placed in research of recent years are discussed elsewhere in this book by Doctors Muir, Ehrlich, Maroudas and Lust. In considering biochemical factors of aetiological importance I will concentrate briefly upon a few topics which are seldom discussed, especially bony remodelling and cartilage mineralisation.

TABLE I   BIOCHEMICAL AETIOLOGICAL FACTORS IN OSTEOARTHRITIS

Secondary Forms of Osteoarthritis

1. Heritable forms
   a. Ehlers-Danlos syndrome (collagen peptide polymorphism), ligamentous laxity.
   b. Abnormal bony and consequently altered articular contours, e.g. Marfan's syndrome or Ollier's disease − with gibbus deformity of spine, etc.

2. Metabolic disorders
   a. Ochronosis − pigment = oxidised homogenetic acid.
   b. Acromegaly − excessive growth hormone and subsequent somatomedin perfusion of tissues leads to bone and cartilage hyperplasia and hypertrophy hypothetically, also leads probably to maldistribution of weight-bearing forces and possibly impaired tissue quality.
   c. Gout, hyperparathyroidism, Paget's disease − direct damage of tophi, subchondral cysts, and Pagetoid lesions, respectively, to bony support of articular cartilage. Possibly deranged metabolism in cartilage cells, especially gout and hyperparathyroidism.

Multiple Aetiological Factors

First of all, when one discusses the biochemical aetiology of osteoarthritis, it is apparent that it is virtually impossible that one factor or even a group of factors will be found responsible (Tables I and II). It is probable that with increased information, primary osteoarthritis will become subdivided on the basis of

TABLE II PRIMARY OSTEOARTHRITIS (Hypothetical)

1. Selective prenatal and developmental errors
   a. Abnormal or 'unequal' growth plate function, e.g. in hip, acetabulum and tibial plateau.
   b. Insoluble collagen crosslinking increased.
   c. Errors of proteoglycan, collagen or other protein synthesis.
   d. Tertiary structural or more complex error of fibril organisation, defective PG aggregation.

2. Cell abiotrophic or senescent changes
   a. b – d above.
   b. Disorder of systems involved in enzymatic degradation of matrix, e.g. proteoglycanases, collagenase.
   c. Calcification disorders — subchondral capillary invasion, expansion of calcified cartilage zone, extension of mineral to synovial fluid and membranes.
   d. Release of lipids, membranes, formation of free radicals.
   e. Altered sensitivity of cells (via receptors) to systemic hormones (e.g. somatomedin, sex hormones, corticosteroids) or local factors (CTAP).
   f. Altered cell biological functions, e.g. phagocytosis, cell death and autolysis.

multiple aetiologies interlinking biochemical and genetic factors. In general, one group of investigators has regarded human ageing cartilage as a successful biomaterial, intrinsically stable biochemically, but reacting to various abusive forces by producing degenerative as well as hypertrophic changes. In contrast, other investigators have viewed cartilage as a dynamic biochemical organ with sensitive responses conditioned by genetic and environmental influences. The role of physical factors in their view is relegated to that of precipitating agents. Such genetic and environmental factors could influence the development of disease a) prenatally, b) during development and maturation, or c) during ageing. It seems likely to the author that both views are correct for some proportion of osteoarthritic patients with considerable overlapping. The problem of whether cartilage fibrillation is simply a consequence of ageing or part of the pathology of progressive osteoarthritic ulceration is also an important aetiological consideration, but beyond the scope of this paper (see Maroudas and Kempson, 1975).

Altered Chondrocyte Function

Some leads as to possible biochemical factors of aetiological importance in osteoarthritis of the primary type may be hidden within the realm of the secondary osteoarthritides (Table I). For example, it has been speculated that minor biochemical developmental errors of growth or remodelling of bone and cartilage during ageing (Harris, 1975) might contribute to primary osteoarthritis in such joints as the hips and knees. Secondly, the increasing data accumulated on altered biomaterial properties of cartilage with ageing must have some biochemical explanation. This explanation may reside in the nature of altered proteoglycans, surface cartilage collagen or deep collagen networks, (Meachim and Freeman, 1973; Maroudas and Kempson, 1975). On the other hand, the author

94

retains a key interest in the hypothesis that there is an increase of irreducible crosslinks in articular collagen as a function of ageing with unfavourable effects on biomechanical properties. Unfortunately, such irreducible crosslinks cannot be currently measured. Studies of reducible crosslinks have failed so far to suggest an increase in numbers as a function of ageing (Jayson et al, 1974). Another topic of revitalised interest is the possible generation of superoxides by ageing cartilage cells with a possible effect of free radical formation on collagen cross-linking. Recent evidence obtained in vitro indicates that such superoxides can degrade proteoglycans (Greenwald et al, 1976) as well as hyaluronic acid, but their presence in vivo in cartilage has not been studied to the author's knowledge. Other functions of chondrocytes have also eluded satisfactory investigation. The phenomena of chondrocytic phagocytosis and chondrocyte autolysis have been discussed, but their possible role in production of focal degradative lesions is just beginning to be studied. In the phagocytic process, one could postulate that lysosomes released into the cartilage might initiate subsurface degradation. Alternatively, during lapses of surface cell membranes in the process of phago-cytosis a sort of extrusion of proteases through the gaps has also to be considered (Reynolds and Werb, 1975). Immunolocalisation studies by Poole, et al, (1974), indicate that cathepsin D is located not only in cells but in the surrounding matrix of animal cartilage. Further evidence that there may be release of unfavourable cellular products in the environment of chondrocytes as a function of ageing has been the finding of vesicles surrounding cells (Ali and Bayliss, 1974; Weiss 1973) and accumulation of lipids in cartilage matrix as a function of ageing (Bonner and Jonnson, 1975). Vesicles in many non-articular cartilaginous sites have been associated with calcification (reviewed by Howell and Pita, 1976), with the presence of acid phosphatase (Thyberg et al, 1973) and with collagenase in vesicles of dentinal matrix (Sorgente and Slavkin, 1977). Research on such topics has been hampered by the lack of our knowledge concerning normal enzymatic machinery of chondrocyte function. Response pathways of synthetic processes, phagocytosis and cell division involve cell membrane receptors affected by physical stimuli, matrix end products and hormones. We need to know a lot more about the role of these receptors, their response to such factors as connective tissue activating peptide, CTAP (Castor 1975), somatomedin B and C (Van Wyk 1973) and pituitary growth factors studied by C Malemud and L Soko-loff (1977). The state of mediation between receptors and pre- and post-transla-tional control of chondrocytic functions still remains more or less a 'black box'. Much more research is needed to define a role in chondrocyte metabolism of prostaglandins, probably of the E, F, G and H series, thromboxanes and cyclic nucleotides (Hamberg et al, 1976).

Cartilage Calcification

The role that cartilage calcification may play in the pathogenesis of osteoarthritis has been previously considered (Howell et al, 1976). It is timely both for reasons of personal research interest and because of recent findings in respect to crystal synovitis associated with osteoarthritis, to consider this again. The author's laboratory has been concerned for years in the basic physiological mechanisms of growth plate calcification as well as in the human disease, chondrocalcinosis. These interests led, as will be discussed below, to a study of metabolic alterations in osteoarthritis related to calcification.

Dieppe et al (1977) have recently proposed an aetiological role for disturbed mineralisation in the clinical picture of osteoarthritis. In the patients with sub-acute or acute synovitis and osteoarthritis studied by Dieppe et al (1977) the aspirated knee effusions showed that a calcium phosphate mineral was a major component of the solid phase of the pellet on centrifugation. Inflammatory cells were also present. Similar clinical findings were also reported by Schumacher et al (1976) in patients with what appeared to be primary osteoarthritis. Stimulated by these findings, Schumacher and his group also injected dogs intra-articularly with a solution containing synthetic calcium phosphate of the apatite class. The mineral caused swelling and heat in the dog joints similar to crystal synovitis caused by calcium pyrophosphate. Based on such findings, it is certainly enter-taining to speculate on a possible metabolic defect in respect to calcification in some of these patients. One can envisage a situation analogous to calcium pyrophosphate deposition disease in which the primary error is believed to rest with the chondrocytes (at least in most cases of chondrocalcinosis) with sporadic leakage into synovial fluid causing the crystal synovitis. At such an early stage of research, one can only consider these studies provocative and important in respect to stimulating much further scrutiny of calcification mechanisms in cartilage. Most previous biochemical data has not supported the assertion that mineralisa-tion has any role in the pathogenesis or aetiology of osteoarthritis (Tables I and II).

Chondrocalcinosis

The author prefers to approach the aetiology of osteoarthritis through considera-tion of a disease in which there clearly is disturbed cartilage mineral metabolism, namely, chondrocalcinosis of the non-familial form seen in middle and old age and described in relationship to pseudogout by McCarty et al (1962). Theories developed on the nature of this disease probably bear to some extent on mechanisms that might be operative at least in a limited degree in osteoarthritis.

The remainder of this article will be devoted to some amplification of these ideas and to possible analogies to be gleaned from survey of this latter disorder.

First of all, chondrocalcinosis exhibits several features that seem to distinguish it from ordinary primary osteoarthritis: 1) specific layering of $CaP_2O_7.2H_2O$ (CPPD) in transitional and upper radial zone articular cartilage clearly visible on roentgenograms, the CPPD being identified by x-ray diffraction or polarized light microscopy in joint tissues and synovial fluid (McCarty, 1977); 2) mineral deposition in cartilage of multiple bones in the wrists, elbows and other joints rarely afflicted with primary osteoarthritis; 3) osteoarthritis often follows rather than precedes detectable mineral deposition; about 2/3 of McCarty's series had accompanying clinically expressed osteoarthritis, usually in knees and hips. Osteoarthritis may also appear in secondary forms of chondrocalcinosis associated with hyperparathyroidism, haemochromatosis etc (McCarty, 1977). It has been postulated that biomechanical properties of the cartilage are reduced by chondrocalcinosis; access of chondrocytes to nutrients might be impaired and cells irritated by the mineral deposits. More hard data to back these possibilities is needed.

It seems that primary osteoarthritis is not related to classical chondrocalcinosis per se. In particular, the studies of Dieppe et al (1977) and Schumacher et al (1976) on patients with primary osteoarthritis showed evidence of what was probably hydroxyapatite in their synovial fluid without CPPD. When human osteoarthritic cartilage was studied by Bollet and Nance (1966) only small amounts of mineral could be found in the cartilage, inasmuch as ash content of articular cartilage above the calcified band attached to bone was very low. X-ray microradiography of osteoarthritic hips in serial sections also failed to show rims of mineral around chondrocytes and only rare deposits in studies by Sokoloff (1977). Admittedly, small amounts of highly labile noncrystalline calcium pyrophosphate in the nascent mineral phase associated with specific clusters of cartilage cells might well be washed out of articular cartilage and not register in gross biochemical cartilage analyses. Detection of early or labile mineral phase has been a problem in research on cartilage growth plate cell biology for decades. Favouring the presence of a mineral disturbance in primary osteoarthritic cartilage was the finding of positive silver nitrate stains over scattered perichondral areas when the block impregnation method of Kashiwa was used to prevent loss of labile phosphates in a small series of osteoarthritic cartilages (Howell and Pita, 1977), and the finding of random CPPD or other crystals under polarising light microscopy in similar cartilage observed histologically by Bjelle (1972).

Pyrophosphate and Mineralisation

As previously mentioned the source of mineral in chondrocalcinosis was postulated to result from abnormal production of CPPD in the matrix under the influence of chondrocytes which normally do not induce calcification. When such cells or similar ones in open growth plates form mineral, it matures to a prototype of hydroxyapatite $Ca_5 (PO_4)_3(OH)$. Thus the presence of CPPD as the sole mineral found in chondrocalcinosis must be explained. The current author among others has been interested in the possibility that pyrophosphate ion is in some manner an intermediate in normal mineral formation in growth cartilage. Cartier and Picard (1956) showed much more efficient uptake of $^{32}PO_4$ into mineral with sheep growth plate slices incubated in vitro with organic agents such as ATP than equivalent concentrations of inorganic phosphate. They postulated that such compounds might be the normal substrates for hydrolytic enzyme release or transfer pyrophosphate into initial mineral phases. If this view were true for pyrophosphate as a precursor ion, then chondrocalcinosis could be due to various metabolic blocks involving failure of hydrolysis of pyrophosphate to phosphate mineral forms (Howell et al, 1975). It was shown that synthetic 'amorphous' or an early calcium phosphate form adsorbed a carbonyl analogue of pyrophosphate, P-C-P (sodium etidronate) which blocked normal transformation of amorphous mineral to hydroxyapatite in vitro at 10^{-4}M (Francis, 1969). Evidence reviewed by Termine (1972) showed kinetic evidence of similar block in such transformation caused by pyrophosphate per se. It seems reasonable from the studies of Fleisch and Neuman (1961) that low concentrations of CPPD might become incorporated on early mineral phases in sites of normal mineral growth, as in cartilage septa, and help control or inhibit mineral growth. Removal of inhibition would be regulated by enzymatic hydrolysis of the pyrophosphate in the environment of the mineral particle. At sites of failure of hydrolysis, intermediate levels of pyrophosphate might help simply to prevent transition to apatite and crystal growth. In the presence of high local levels of pyrophosphate, not only would the apatite mineral form not grow, but CPPD could conceivably precipitate at neutral pH and accrue crystals of the type seen in chondrocalcinosis. An alternative view postulates need for a special nucleating mould on which CPPD specifically grows either in cartilage or synovial membrane. This latter view is still quite possible but has no relevant supporting data known to the author.

The view fostered in the author's personal work would favour pyrophosphate from cartilage cells at sites of calcification in growth plates with its hydrolysis in the ultramicro environment of the expanding apatite mineral phase (Howell et al, 1975). This hydrolysis is favoured by the fact that no additional pyrophosphate to that which could be adsorbed from lymph was found in a study of cartilage septa by Wuthier et al, (1972). The concept would predict a failure of pyrophosphate hydrolysis in the ultramicro environment of new mineral phase in chondrocalcinosis, together with excessive accumulation of pyrophosphate surrounding new CPPD mineral clusters.

Evidence that some biochemical reaction of this sort might actually occur in chondocalcinosis comes from the finding that pyrophosphate ion concentration is highly significantly elevated in the synovial fluid but not in the serum or the urine. The findings of Russell et al (1970) have been amply confirmed and strongly suggest a local metabolic disorder of pyrophosphate metabolism. One alternative view that there might be a failure of synovial fluid pyrophosphatase to degrade normal output of pyrophosphate by joint tissues seems interdicted by careful studies by McCarty (1977) in which the proportion of pyrophosphate in human synovial fluid removed by endogenous phosphatases in vitro was only an insignificant fraction of that turned over by efflux into lymph and venous blood. Furthermore, no error of red cell phosphatase was found in chondrocalcinosis so that a systemic genetic defect of phosphatase in the disease seems unlikely (McCarty and Pepe, 1972). Thus, the accumulation of CPPD in articular cartilage in chondrocalcinosis seems to result from a switching-on of mineral-forming function. Some evidence that this type of induction is possible was shown in cartilage cells in vitro by Urist et al, (1975) with bone morphogenetic factor, identified so far as a polypeptide which Urist believes is attached to bone collagen; one must also postulate a superimposed defect of pyrophosphate hydrolysis whereby the 'wrong' mineral if formed.

Mineral Metabolism in Osteoarthritis

Pyrophosphate metabolism may be relevant to primary osteoarthritis to the extent that, even without chondrocalcinosis on x-ray, 17 patients with primary osteoarthritis showed a disturbance of cartilage behaviour which the author construed as evidence for switched-on mineral formation (Howell et al, 1975). In these patients cartilage was obtained at surgery of the knee and hip, and the pieces of diced cartilage (after cleaning and dissection) were incubated in Eagle's basal medium. The samples elaborated pyrophosphate into the medium, in contrast to cartilage from patients with avascular necrosis, rheumatoid arthritis and femoral neck fracture; all controls without signs of additional osteoarthritis. Furthermore, a highly significant elevation of pyrophosphate was found in the synovial fluid of such patients compared to normal and rheumatoid controls. It was noted by Silcox and McCarty (1974), who confirmed the above findings, that only patients with ulcerated cartilage had high pyrophosphate levels in the synovial fluid. We also found that only ulcerated osteoarthritic cartilage showed significant pyrophosphate elaboration on incubation in vitro. Cartilage from two cases of overt chondrocalcinosis displayed high rates of pyrophosphate output into Eagle's basal medium; sufficient if extrapolated to total cartilage in the knee to account for the total turnover of pyrophosphate in chondrocalcinosis in the knees of patients studied by McCarty (1977).

Evidence that this is not a function of cell proliferation or matrix synthesis came from studies of rabbit cartilage growth plates and rabbit ear cartilage on three month old animals. Brisk cell division and matrix synthesis proceeds in the ear cartilage as well as upper articular cartilage of normal rabbits as shown by thymidine uptake over cells, but only the microdissected hypertrophic and proliferating cell cartilage of the epiphyseal island and of the growth plate elaborated pyrophosphate (Howell et al, 1976). Pyrophosphate output could not be suppressed by colchicine or actinomycin D and other controls, such as a lack of output of lactic dehydrogenase, indicated cell lysis was not a likely explanation. We postulated that the pyrophosphate output was specifically related to the mechanisms of normal calcification in the rabbit growth plate. Growth in cell cultures has been studied by Lust et al, (1976). These authors found that cultured chondrocytes failed to put out pyrophosphate into the

99

TABLE III   HYPOTHESIS ON THE AETIOLOGY OF NONFAMILIAL
CHONDROCALCINOSIS AND SECONDARY OSTEOARTHRITIS

Cartilage cells

Senescence, abiotrophy — genetic factors

Inductive mechanism for
cartilage calcification

↓   Access of mineral to joint space with
Chondrocalcinosis   → sporadic inflammatory attacks

↓

Poor resistance to
physical forces
↓
Cartilage ulceration
↓
Joint remodelling
↓
Widened layer of calcified, and
narrowed layer of uncalcified
cartilage facing joint space

surrounding medium under any conditions. My interpretation of their results is
that the mechanisms for calcification have been switched off in the course of
this type of in vitro cell culturing. However, they demonstrated brisk cell division
and matrix synthesis by different cultures of human osteoarthritic and chondro-
calcinotic chondrocytes. This finding would strongly indicate that these functions
per se are not associated with extracellular elaboration of pyrophosphate. Perhaps
release is associated with the metabolism of nucleotides such as ATP or related
precursors. Nucleotide content was found increased in the growth plate matrix
in expressed fluid from growth cartilage by Wuthier, (1977), as well as in aspirated
fluid by micropuncture from growth plates in vivo studied by Howell et al, (1968).
Direct analysis of pyrophosphate in puncture fluid has not been possible in our
laboratory due to a high background of interfering fluorescent compounds.

Criticism of this viewpoint arises in some obvious ways. If pyrophosphate is
elaborated by cells locally as a precursor, how does it get through the cell
membrane? Pyrophosphate fails, notoriously, to be transported through intact
limiting cell membranes (Russell, 1976). Answers to these questions require a
brief perusal of the cellular mechanisms currently believed to be involved in
normal calcification.

If matrix vesicles are the normal site of new mineral formation and not
adventitious landmarks of cell degeneration, pyrophosphate could be extruded
during the exocytotic pinching off of filopodia of cartilage cells, believed
generally to be the source of these midseptal vesicles (Rabinovitch and Anderson,
1976). The pyrophosphate might be extruded complexed to some agent or simply
leaked out as an ion at the time of membrane discontinuity. Alternatively,
formation of 3.5 cyclic AMP in the cell membrane from ATP in response to

100

extracellular regulators of chondrocyte function might liberate pyrophosphate into the external environment rather than into the cell; but no data exists on this point. Thirdly, the membrane of distal hypertrophic cartilage cells, and perhaps articular cells induced to mineralise might accumulate metabolic products which alter membrane permeability. It was shown by Wuthier (1971) that a striking rise of lysophospholipids normally accumulated as a product of activation of endogenous phospholipase A in the cartilage of this distal growth plate. These products, added to cartilage cells in vivo, can alter the cell's permeability to ions (Wuthier, 1977). Both proteoglycans (Smith, 1970) and collagen in bone minera-lising sites (Glimcher, 1977) have been suggested as alternative foci for nucleation. This same mechanism might apply regardless of the final sequence of nucleation.

The critical feature that the various alternative views of the final apparatus for mineral generation have in common is a defective pyrophosphatase and possibly nucleotidase function to deliver phosphate into nucleating sites, whatever these be. Articular cartilage has been reported to store calcium excessively (Maroudas, 1976). Certainly a glycoprotein described by de Bernard and Vittur, (1973) in cartilage, and the carboxyglutamic acid containing protein isolated from bone, (Hauschka et al, 1975) dentine and other tissue are candidates for the calcium-storing function in a proteoglycan or collagen complex nucleator. On the other hand, the same or similar proteins or phospholipids (Boskey and Posner 1975) in the membranes might bind and store calcium in a postulated matrix vesicle nucleator. Cartilage fluid obtained by micro-puncture (Howell et al, 1968) in rats, and whole cartilage electrolyte profiles in puppies (Eichelberger and Roma, 1954) and in calves (Howell et al, 1960) revealed calcium storage prior to calcification. The need for a phosphatase is supported by further data relating to normal calcification obtained from micropuncture fluids (Howell et al, 1977).

Should 'hard data' emerge showing that a failure of pyrophosphatase-nucleo-tidase function definitely caused CPPD mineral deposition and high synovial fluid pyrophosphate, what relationship does this have to the findings of high pyro-phosphate concentrations in osteoarthritic synovial fluid, and output of pyro-phosphate by osteoarthritic cartilage in vitro? Obviously, we do not know. A working hypothesis has already been outlined, indicating a role for pyrophos-phate in normal calcification. Possibly in osteoarthritis without CPPD deposition, there is a different type of new mineral deposition. Such is the formation of hydroxyapatite in the very deepest layers of the articular cartilage just on the edge of the calcified cartilage, induced by unknown factors related to sub-chondral bony remodelling.

Remodelling of Bone

Preliminary evidence has been found for subchondral remodelling at weight bearing sites in the knees and hips of humans analysed as a function of ageing (Lane et al, 1975). New capillary penetration to the tidemark, tidemark reduplication and remodelling of subchondral bone with fresh calcification along the invading vessels seemed to indicate a reopened growth plate function. Since this process became increasingly prevalent per unit area of cartilage as a function of ageing after age 50 years in humans, it raises the question of a possible aetiological role in osteoarthritis. Other factors (Table III) may also bear on this problem. Once osteoarthritis develops, subchondral bony remodelling probably intensifies and many sites in hips and knees appear to have thinned articular cartilage with a thickened region of calcified cartilage and bone beneath.

In view of the findings of Lane et al, (1975), this reviewer would propose the hypothesis that 1) at least in most cases of primary osteoarthritis subchondral remodelling occurs in high frequency, especially at weight-bearing sites; 2) mid-layer cartilage over such sites sporadically undergoes changes which induce mineral formation as a result of failure of environmental pyrophosphatase to abort the normal mineral forming response to pyrophosphate; 3) at times when pyrophosphatase activity is adequate to inhibit CPPD formation, new hydroxyapatite mineral might form in the ulcerated osteoarthritic cartilage, as observed by Ali and Bayliss (1974), prior to inducing the inflammatory synovial fluids seen by Dieppe et al, (1977), and Schumacher, (1976).

The high frequency of these events is reinforced by the prevalence of a high synovial fluid pyrophosphate (Altman et al, 1973), elevated alkaline phosphatase in osteoarthritic cartilage (Ali and Bayliss, 1974) and histologic localisation of alkaline phosphatase (Stockwell and Meachim, 1973) in ageing rabbit chondrocytes in the radial zone adjacent to calcified cartilage.

Nevertheless in the light of current knowledge one must take the view that such disturbances involving mineral metabolism are probably not of aetiological importance but constitute a variable feature of the pathogenetic processes. One can but hope that with improved understanding of the metabolism of normal and degenerate articular cartilage a sector of the primary osteoarthritic population will be delineated in which there is an underlying disturbance of mineral metabolism.

References

Ali SY, Bayliss MT (1974) In *Normal and Osteoarthrotic Articular Cartilage*. Eds. SY Ali, MW Elves and DH Leaback, Institute of Orthopaedics, Stanmore, University of London, p. 189

Altman RD, Muniz OE, Pita JC (1973) *Arthritis and Rheumatism, 16,* 171

Benderley, H and Maroudas A (1975) In *Symposium on Cartilage, Annals of the Rheumatic Diseases, 34,* Supplement 2

Bjelle AO (1972) *Annals of the Rheumatic Diseases 31,* 449; and (1977) *Personal communication*

Bollet AJ and Nance JL (1966) *Journal of Clinical Investigation, 45,* 1170

Bonner WM, Jonsson H, Malanos C et al (1975) *Arthritis and Rheumatism 18,* 461

Boskey AL and Posner AS (1975) *Calcified Tissue Research, 19,* 283

Cartier P and Picard J (1956) *Bulletin de la Societe de Chimie Biologique 38,* 707

Castor CW (1975) *Presentation at VIII European Rheumatology Congress, Helsinki, Finland* de Bernard B and Vittur F (1973) In *Proceedings of the International Colloquium on Physical Chemistry and Crystallography of Apatites of Biological Interest*, Paris, France, Centre National de la Recherche Scientifique. Ed: G Montel

Dieppe PA, Huskisson EC, Crocker PR and Willoughby DA (1976) *Lancet, i*, 266

Eichelberger L and Roma M (1954) *American Journal of Physiology 178*, 296

Fleisch H and Neuman WF (1961) *American Journal of Physiology 200*, 1296

Francis MD (1969) *Calcified Tissue Research 3*, 151

Glimcher MJ (1976) In *Handbook of Physiology VII Endocrinology*. Eds. RO Greep and EB Astwood, Washington, American Physiological Society, p.25

Greenwald RA, Moy WW and Lazarus D (1976) *Arthritis and Rheumatism 19*, 799

Hamberg M, Svensson J and Samuelsson B (1976) In *Advances in Prostaglandin and Thromboxane Research*, Eds. B Samuelsson and R Paoletti, Raven Press, New York, p.19

Harris WH (1975) In *Proceedings of 3rd Open Scientific Meeting of the Hip Society*, CV Mosby, St Louis

Hauschka PV, Lian JB and Gallop PM (1975) *Proceedings of the National Academy of Sciences, 72*, 3925

Howell DS, Delchamps E, Riemer W and Kiem I (1960) *Journal of Clinical Investigation, 39*, 919

Howell DS, Pita JC, Marquez JF and Madruga JE (1968) *Journal of Clinical Investigation, 47*, 1121

Howell DS, Muniz OE, Pita JC and Enis JE (1975) *Journal of Clinical Investigation, 56*, 1473

Howell DS and Pita JC (1976) *Clinical Orthopaedics 118*, 208

Howell DS, Sapolsky AI, Pita JC and Woessner JF (1976) *Seminars in Arthritis and Rheumatism, 5*, 365

Howell DS, Muniz OE, Pita JC and Enis JE (1976) *Arthritis and Rheumatism, 19*, 488

Howell DS, Pita JC and Muniz OE (1977) *Journal of Dental Research 56A*, A105

Howell DS and Pita JC (1977) Unpublished observations

Jayson MIV, Herbert CM and Bailey AJ (1974) In *Normal and Osteoarthrotic Articular Cartilage*. Eds. SY Ali, MW Elves and DH Leaback, Institute of Orthopaedics, University of London, Stanmore, p. 219

Lane LB, Villacin A and Bullough PG (1975) *Journal of Bone and Joint Surgery, 57*, 576

Lust G, Nuki G and Seegmiller JE (1976) *Arthritis and Rheumatism 19*, 479

Maroudas A and Kempson GE (1975) *Symposium on Cartilage, Annals of the Rheumatic Disease 34*, Supplement 2

McCarty DJ, Kohn NN and Faires JS (1962) *Annals of Internal Medicine 56*, 711

McCarty DJ and Pepe PF (1972) *Journal of Laboratory and Clinical Medicine 79*, 277

McCarty DJ (1976) *Proceedings of the Conference on Pseudogout and Pyrophosphate Metabolism, Santa Ynez, CA, October 1975. Arthritis and Rheumatism, 19*, Supplement 3

McCarty DJ (1976) *Arthritis and Rheumatism 19*, 275

Meachim G and Freeman MAR (1973) In *Adult Articular Cartilage*, Isaac Pitman & Sons, Oxford, p.287

Poole AR, Hembry RM and Dingle JT (1974) *Journal of Cell Science 14*, 139

Rabinovitch AL and Anderson HC (1976) *Federation Proceedings 35*, 112

Reynolds JJ and Werb Z (1975) In *Extracellular Matrix Influences on Gene Expression*. Eds. HC Slavkin and RC Greulich, Academic Press, New York, p.225

Russell RGG, (1976) *Arthritis and Rheumatism 19*, 465

Schumacher HR, Tse R, Reginato A, Miller J and Maurer K (1976) *Arthritis and Rheumatism 19*, 821

Silcox DC and McCarty DJ (1974) *Journal of Laboratory and Clinical Medicine 83*, 518

Sorgente, N and Slavkin, HC, Brownell AG, (1976) *Journal of Cell Biology 70*, 271

Smith JW (1970) *Journal of Cell Science 6*, 843

Sokoloff L (1977) Personal communication

Stockwell RA and Meachim G (1973) In *Adult Articular Cartilage*. Ed. MAR Freeman, Isaac Pitman & Sons, Oxford, p.51

Termine JD (1972) *Clinical Orthopaedics 85*, 207

Thyberg J, Lohmander S and Friberg U (1973) *Journal of Ultrastructure Research 45*, 407

Urist MR, Nogami H and Terashima Y (1975) In *Extracellular Matrix Influences on Gene Expression,* Eds. HC Slavkin and RC Greulich, Academic Press, New York. p.609

Van Wyk JJ, Underwood LE, Lister RC and Marshall RN (1973) *American Journal of Diseases of Childhood. 126,* 705

Weiss C (1973) *Federation Proceedings 32,* 1459

Wuthier RE (1971) *Calcified Tissue Research 8,* 36

Wuthier RE Bisaz S, Russell RGG and Fleisch H (1972) *Calcified Tissue Research 10,* 198

Wuthier RE (1977) Personal communication

11

MINERAL-CONTAINING MATRIX VESICLES IN HUMAN OSTEOARTHROTIC CARTILAGE

S Yousuf Ali

Introduction

Biochemical analysis of human osteoarthrotic cartilage and its comparison with normal articular cartilage had led us to postulate a calcification abnoramlity in the diseased tissue (Ali & Evans, 1973a). In the light of our newer knowledge of the mechanism of initial calcification in growth cartilage (Ali et al, 1970; Ali & Evans, 1973b; Ali, 1976; Anderson, 1976) it was decided to re-evaluate the ultrastructural and enzymic aspects of human articular cartilage to see if there was any evidence of abnormal mineralisation in osteoarthrosis (Ali & Bayliss, 1974; Ali & Wisby, 1975; Ali & Wisby, 1976). LC Johnson (1962) and others had suggested that the remodelling of subchondral bone could be an aetiological factor in osteoarthrosis; McCarty (1970) included in his concept of 'crystal deposition disease' the likelihood that apatite and other related crystals could be a source of inflammation and arthritis. Recently, Dieppe et al (1976) have reported the presence of hydroxyapatite nodules in the synovial fluid of arthritic patients. The morphological and chemical similarity of the synovial fluid apatite particles to the apatite crystal nodules that we have observed in articular cartilage is so close (Ali, 1977) that we feel they probably originate in articular cartilage through the calcification process initiated by matrix vesicles. It is the purpose of this chapter to firstly review the ultrastructural observations in articular cartilage which pointed to the presence of extracellular particles ; secondly, to summarise our present knowledge of the mechanism of initial calcification in epiphyseal cartilage; thirdly to present evidence to suggest that the matrix vesicles in articular cartilage are functionally similar to those in the growth cartilage, and, finally, to interpret the data as a means of providing a new concept for the pathogenesis of one form of osteoarthrosis.

Ultrastructure of Articular Cartilage

Early electron microscope observations of rabbit articular cartilage had shown a pericellular distribution of electron-dense lipidic debris in the matrix surrounding the chondrocytes (Barnett et al, 1963). The debris was found to contain rounded bodies (up to 200 nm in diameter) which sometimes had a granular appearance and their accumulation in articular cartilage was age related. Both fibrillated and non-fibrillated specimens of human articular cartilage showed similar electron-dense membranous particles surrounding healthy cells and it was suggested that these were derived from cytoplasmic processes extending from the chondrocyte into the surrounding matrix (Ghadially et al, 1965; Ghadially & Roy, 1969). Meachim (1969) found them in human osteoarthrotic articular cartilage, and their distribution appeared similar to the distribution of phospholipid and neutral lipid by light microscopic histochemistry by Stockwell (1965). Similar vesicular bodies were seen in other studies of articular cartilage and they have been variously described as cellular debris (Ruettner & Spycher, 1968), Corona vesicles (Spycher et al, 1969), matrix granules (Zimny & Redler, 1969), membranous debris (Ghadially et al, 1971), lipid material (Silberberg & Hasler, 1968), and extracellular lipid (Weiss & Mirow, 1972). The function of these pericellular bodies has not been satisfactorily explained. Initially, Ghadially et al (1965) considered these osmiophilic bodies to consist of physiologically extruded lipid from the cells. Chrisman et al (1967), using electron histochemical methods, showed the presence of esterase and cathepsin-type of activity in the extracellular particles in articular cartilage and thought of them as lysosomes. Bonner and Owen (1969) in an abstract mentioned that these bodies stained with lipid stains and at electron microscopic level reacted with substrates for acid phosphatase, β-glucuronidase and n-acetyl-beta-glucosaminidase. They too postulated them as extracellular lysosomes but, to date, none of the pictures or evidence has been published in detail. Thyberg and Friberg (1972) using epiphyseal cartilage showed some acid phosphatase and aryl sulphatase activity to be associated with extracellular vesicles.

Calcification of Epiphyseal Cartilage

It is only recently that the sequence of biochemical events responsible for the mineralisation of growth cartilage and its subsequent transformation into cancellous bone have been partially elucidated, largely through ultrastructural studies. Bonucci (1967) and Anderson (1969) demonstrated that the longitudinal septa of epiphyseal cartilage contain extracellular membranous matrix vesicles (100 nm in diameter) which display the first microcrystals of hydroxyapatite. Similar matrix vesicles or dense bodies have been found in a variety of mineralising tissues, such as medullary bone, dentin, calcifying aorta, and antler horns (see review by Anderson, 1976). Electron histochemistry demonstrated the presence of alkaline phosphatase in these vesicles but no acid phosphatase (Matsuzawa & Anderson, 1971). Biochemical isolation and characterisation has shown that matrix vesicles contain most of the alkaline phosphatase, pyrophosphatase and

ATPase activity of growth cartilage and that they are derived from the cell processes of chondrocytes and are not lysosomes (Ali et al, 1970; Ali, 1976). The mechanism by which matrix vesicles concentrate calcium to induce apatite formation has been studied by using isotopes, especially [45] calcium, and it is clear that calcium can bind to the membranes of the vesicles or diffuse passively into the lumen under physiological conditions. In the presence of low calcium concentration, and an energy supply (ATP), they can actively take in calcium against a concentration gradient (Ali & Evans, 1973b; Ali, 1976; Ali et al, 1977). Systematic electron probe analysis of a single longitudinal septum of epiphyseal cartilage has established the sequence of how matrix vesicles take in, first calcium and then phosphorous, to form crystals of apatite which then grow to form mineral nodules which subsequently coalesce to form calcified septa (Ali, 1976; Ali et al, 1977). The role of matrix vesicles in various disorders of calcification and growth is under investigation.

Function of Matrix Vesicles in Articular Cartilage

With our knowledge of matrix vesicles in growth cartilage we have re-examined human articular cartilage to see if they play a role in mineralisation of the joint tissue, especially under pathological conditions. Some of this information and most of the technical methods used in this study have been published elsewhere (Ali & Evans, 1973a; Ali & Bayliss, 1974; Ali & Wisby, 1975; Ali, 1976). The questions that needed an answer were: are the matrix vesicles in human articular cartilage similar to those in epiphyseal cartilage, morphologically (that is in size, appearance and distribution), chemically (enzyme content, whether alkaline phosphatase is cellular or extracellular and associated with these vesicles) and functionally (are microcrystals and apatite nodules associated with them)? It was also important to evaluate whether any changes occurred in human arthritic cartilage. Ultrastructural examination of articular cartilage confirmed that the dense bodies surrounding the pericellular area (Figure 3) were very similar to matrix vesicles in growth cartilage (compare Figures 1,2,4,5 and 6). Their appearance showed the same osmiophilic characteristics and their size, which varied from 50 nm to 250 nm in diameter was very similar to the matrix vesicles, although they appeared more heterogenous (Figures 2,4,5 and 6). A double membrane could be seen (Figures 2,4 and 6; see also Ali & Bayliss, 1974; Ali & Wisby, 1975) and the vesicles were present at all levels of the articular cartilage, but were more frequent in the IV zone in the tidemark region adjoining the subchondral bone. In this region microcrystals were present inside the vesicles and mineral nodules could be seen either forming from vesicles or lying next to them (Figures 5 & 6) and this was again very similar to growth cartilage. Obviously, it was not possible at electron microscope level, to put any number to their frequency and occurrence, and we had to turn to biochemistry for quantitation.

Enzymic digestion of human articular cartilage with collagenase and separation of cells from the extracellular fractions has revealed that the major portion

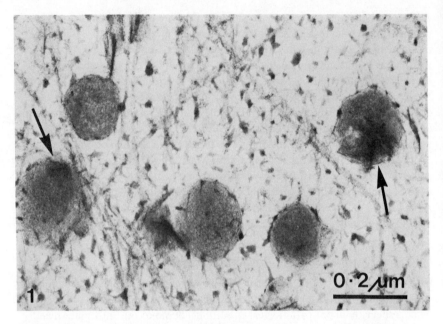

Figure 1. Electron microscope picture of matrix vesicles, some with crystal needles inside them (arrows) are shown in the longitudinal septa matrix in the hypertrophic region of rabbit proximal tibial growth plate. All the electron micrographs are stained with uranyl acetate and lead citrate. Compare these vesicles with those in human articular cartilage in Figures 2, 4, 5 and 6, shown at comparable magnifications. X 100,000

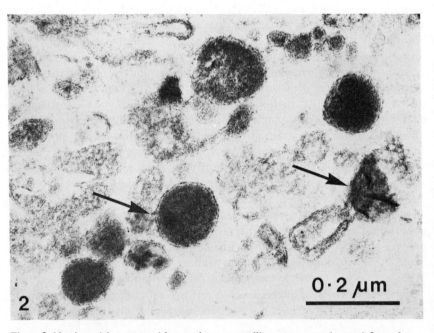

Figure 2. Matrix vesicles, some with granular or crystalline appearance (arrows) from the middle zone of human (age = 25 years) articular osteophyte. Note the double membrane and compare with vesicles shown in other pictures. X 128,000

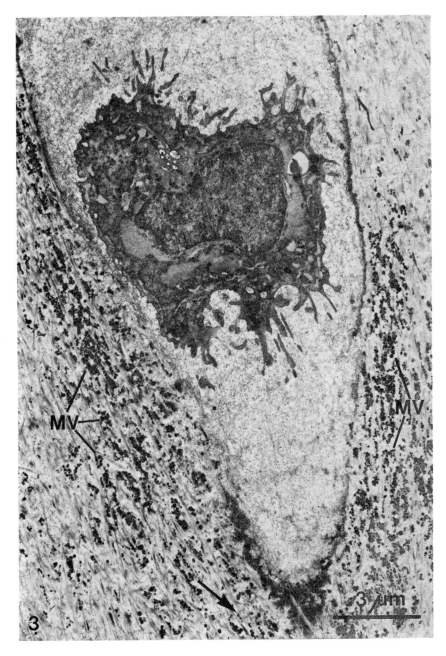

Figure 3. Chondrocyte from the middle zone of adult human (age = 38 years) articular cartilage, showing the pericellular distribution of matrix vesicles (MV) scattered amongst the collagen fibrils. A small area (arrow) is shown at a higher magnification in Figure 4. X 8000

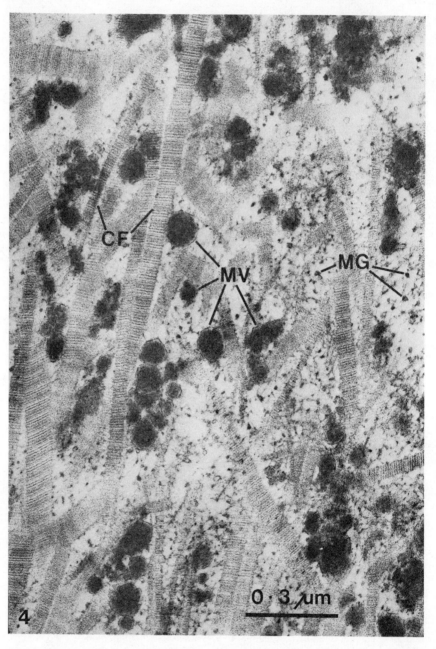

Figure 4. Higher magnification picture of the arrowed area in Figure 3 showing the matrix vesicles (MV) scattered amongst the collagen fibrils (CF) in the pericellular region outside the chondrocyte lacuna, in human (age = 38 years) articular cartilage. The collagen fibrils are thicker than in growth cartilage but the proteoglycan matrix granules (MG) are smaller. X 82,000

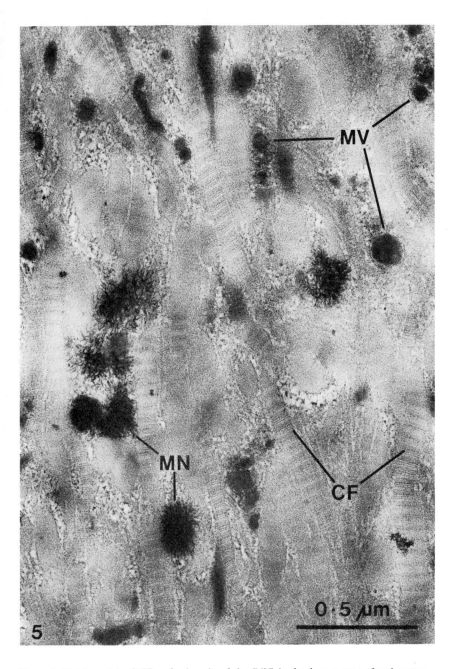

Figure 5. Matrix vesicles (MV) and mineral nodules (MN) in the deeper zone of early osteo-arthrotic human (age = 32 years) articular cartilage. The vesicles have a double membrane and the collagen fibres (CF) are thicker than in the middle zone of articular cartilage and of the growth plate. (Compare with Figure 1.) X 66,000

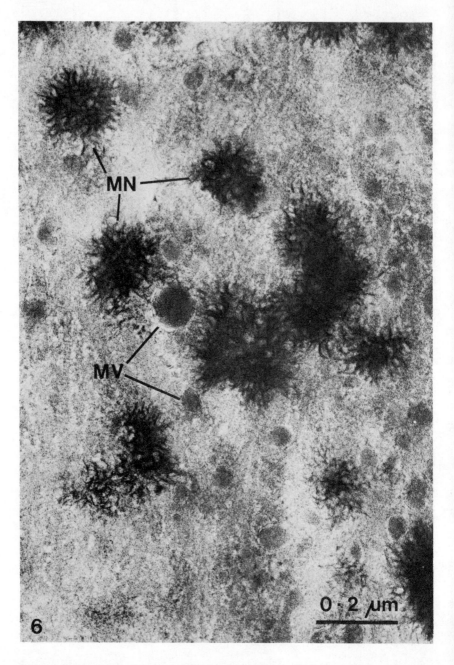

Figure 6. Matrix vesicles (MV) and mineral nodules (MN) from the pericellular region of the deep zone of osteoarthrotic human (age = 32 years) articular cartilage. The matrix vesicles have a double membrane and are closely associated with the apatite-like crystal clusters and nodules. X 112,000

112

of the alkaline phosphatase activity of this tissue is not present in chondrocytes but in the matrix vesicles (Ali, 1976). Indeed the pattern of distribution of this enzyme in the various fractions is indistinguishable from growth cartilage but is quite different to that obtained with elastic ear cartilage or other non-calcifying tissues (Ali, 1976). This indicates that articular cartilage is similar to growth cartilage in this respect. An analysis of the alkaline phosphatase activity levels in normal and osteoarthrotic articular cartilage, from human specimens is shown in Table I. There is high enzyme activity in juvenile and adolescent normal articular cartilage, but this settles down to a low level in adult life. In osteoarthrotic

TABLE I. Comparison of Alkaline Phosphatase Activity in Normal and Osteoarthrotic Human Articular Cartilage (50–80 year group)
The enzyme level is expressed as mg.phosphate/g cartilage from femoral heads.
For further details see Ali and Bayliss (1974)

Cartilage	Number	Mean	SD	P
Normal (Types I and II)	19	0.038	0.031	
				0.01 – 0.001
Osteoarthrotic (Type IV)	23	0.431	0.589	

cartilage, the enzyme level is sometimes thirty times that of the normal in the same age group. This may be an indication that there is an increase in the number of matrix vesicles in osteoarthrotic cartilage, although a specific enzyme increase cannot be ruled out. Ultrastructurally, matrix vesicles were more frequently encountered in the mid-zone of osteoarthrotic cartilage than in the normal (see also Ali & Bayliss, 1974; Ali & Wisby, 1975). They also appeared to be more granular and frequently contained needle-like crystals inside them which were more common in IV zone (Figures 2,5 and 6). In osteoarthrotic cartilage, some mid-zone vesicles also displayed granular or microcrystalline appearance and nodules of apatite-like mineral in the deeper zones (Figures 5 and 6). Osteophytic cartilage, which had high alkaline phosphatase activity also had many granular matrix vesicles (Figure 2).

Implications for the Aetiology of Osteoarthrosis

This electron microscopic and biochemical analysis indicates that the calcification mechanism may be abnormal in osteoarthrotic cartilage and could therefore have serious consequences. Articular cartilage has a great affinity for calcium and has a high calcium content (Eichelberger et al, 1958). An abnormal calcification mechanism can produce cartilage degeneration in a number of ways. For example, if there is an increase in matrix vesicles and mineral nodules in the deeper zones of cartilage, this may lead to focal conversion of the basal portions of the tissue into calcified cartilage and eventually bone. This may alter the 'tidemark' region to reduplication and permit an advance of the mineral front, implying that articular cartilage, which can be considered a latent growth plate, has reverted to a growth phase again. This remodelling near the subchondral bone will put greater pressure on the remaining layer of cartilage which may then become more susceptible to degradation by the normal wear process. This concept fits in very well with that put forward originally by LC Johnson (1962) and others. Moreover, any change in local concentration of calcium in articular cartilage could alter the various physico-chemical properties of the tissue, such as the water binding capacity, the colloidal charge density, the swelling pressure and, thus, the elasticity of the tissue (Gersh & Catchpole, 1960; Sokoloff, 1963; Kempson, 1973; Elmore et al, 1963; Maroudas, 1973). These changes will make the articular cartilage more prone to wear under pressure. In addition, the presence of mineral crystallites and nodules in the middle and upper layers of cartilage will lead to physical, abrasive wear of the whole tissue.

Finally, some of our results with regards to matrix vesicles and the findings of apatite-like crystals and nodules in cartilage can be correlated with some of the implications of crystal-induced inflammation in joints. McCarty (1970) introduced the concept of 'crystal-deposition disease' and found that apart from urate and pyrophosphate deposits, two other crystal types could be found in human articular cartilage and adjoining tissues and fluids, namely hydroxyapatite and dicalcium phosphate dihydrate. Recurrent acute inflammation associated with focal apatite crystal deposition has been found in some patients (McCarty & Gatter, 1966). Dieppe et al (1976) not only analysed and demonstrated hydroxyapatite nodules in synovial fluid, but also showed the inflammatory reaction which the mineral particles could produce. Their work has permitted them to postulate an 'apatite deposition disease' as one form of osteoarthrosis. The particle size described by Dieppe et al (1976) varied from 0.15μm to 0.8μm and the matrix vesicles found by us in human articular cartilage were from 0.05 to 0.25μm, and when nodules were formed from them, the diameter increased to 0.6μm. Thus, the mineral nodules, shown in Figures 5 and 6, are very near in size and description to those shown by Dieppe et al (1976). It would have to be stressed that in normal articular cartilage these mineral nodules associated with the matrix vesicles are commonly found in the deeper layers. It is possible that in osteoarthrotic cartilage they occur in the middle zones and if there were coincident deep fibrillation or vertical clefts in the cartilage, then it is easy to visualise these nodules being shed into the joint cavity and setting up an inflammatory cycle. It should also be stressed that in chondrocalcinosis there appears to be a slight decrease in alkaline phosphatase activity (Reginato et al, 1974) of articular cartilage, whereas we have found an elevation in osteoarthrotic cartilage and our findings are, therefore, quite different to pseudogout. It is easy

114

to see that lack of alkaline phosphatase (pyrophosphatase) will lead to an accumulation of pyrophosphate, whereas increase in alkaline phosphatase will permit the hydrolysis of phosphate-containing substrates (e.g. ATP, PPi, G-6-P, G-1-P, etc) and lead to the formation of apatite (Ali, 1976). Howell et al (1974) have found that articular cartilage is capable of extruding pyrophosphate, especially in some forms of osteoarthrosis. We therefore agree with Dieppe et al (1976) and feel that apatite deposition disease should be added to the crystal deposition diseases defined by McCarty (1970) and suggest that the formation of apatite nodules in cartilage and in synovial fluid is dependent to a large extent on the distribution and function of matrix vesicles.

Acknowledgments

I am grateful to the PF Charitable Trust and the Nuffield Foundation for financial support, and to Angela Wisby for technical help in Electron Microscopy.

References

Ali, SY (1976) *Federation Proceedings, 35,* 135
Ali, SY (1977) In *Perspectives in Inflammation.* (Ed) DA Willoughby. MTP Press, Lancaster. Page 211
Ali, SY and Bayliss, MT (1974) In *Normal and Osteoarthrotic Articular Cartilage.* (Ed) SY Ali, MW Elves and DH Leaback. Institute of Orthopaedics Publication, London. Page 189
Ali, SY and Evans, L (1973a) *Federation Proceedings, 32,* 1494
Ali, SY and Evans, L (1973b) *Biochemical Journal, 134,* 647
Ali, SY, Sajdera, SW and Anderson, HC (1970) *Proceedings of the National Academy of Sciences of the United States of America, 67,* 1513
Ali, SY and Wisby, A (1975) *Annals of the Rheumatic Diseases, 34, Suppt.2,* 21
Ali, SY and Wisby, A (1976) *Proceedings of the Royal Microscopical Society, 11,* 62
Ali, SY, Wisby, A, Evans, L and Craig-Gray, J (1977) *Calcified Tissue Research, 22,* suppl. 490
Anderson, HC (1969) *Journal of Cell Biology, 41,* 59
Anderson, HC (1976) In *The Biochemistry and Physiology of Bone.* (Ed) GH Bourne. Academic Press, New York. Volume IV, Page 135
Barnett, CH, Cochrane, W and Palfrey, AJ (1963) *Annals of the Rheumatic Diseases, 22,* 389
Bonner, WM Jr and Owen, C (1968) *Arthritis and Rheumatism, 11,* 816
Bonucci, E (1967) *Journal of Ultrastructure Research, 20,* 33
Chrisman, OD, Semonsky, C and Beusch, KG (1967) In *The Healing of Osseous Tissue.* (Ed) RA Robinson. National Academy of Science, National Research Council Publication, Washington, DC. Page 169
Dieppe, PA, Huskinsson, EC, Crocker, P and Willoughby, DA (1976) *Lancet, i,* 266
Eichelberger, L, Akeson, WH and Roma, M (1968) *Journal of Bone and Joint Surgery, 40A,* 142
Elmore, SM, Sokoloff, L, Norris, G and Carmeci, P (1963) *Journal of Applied Physiology, 18,* 393
Gersh, I and Catchpole, HR (1960) *Perspectives in Biology and Medicine, 3,* 282
Ghadially, FN, Fuller, JA and Kirkaldy-Willis, WH (1971) *Archives of Pathology, 92,* 356
Ghadially, FN, Meachim, G and Collins, DH (1965) *Annals of the Rheumatic Diseases, 24,* 136
Ghadially, FN and Roy, S (1969) In *Ultrastructure of Synovial Joints in Health and Disease.*

Butterworth, London

Howell, DS, Muniz, O and Pita, JC (1974) In *Normal and Osteoarthrotic Articular Cartilage.* (Ed) SY Ali, MW Elves and DH Leaback. Institute of Orthopaedics Publication, London. Page 177

Johnson, LC (1962) *Journal of the American Veterinary Medical Association, 141,* 1237

Kempson, GE (1973) In *Adult Articular Cartilage.* (Ed) MAR Freeman. Pitman Medical, Tunbridge Wells

Maroudas, A (1973) In *Adult Articular Cartilage.* (Ed) MAR Freeman. Pitman Medical, Tunbridge Wells

Matsuzawa, I and Anderson, HC (1971) *Journal of Histochemistry and Cytochemistry, 19,* 801

McCarty, DJ (1970) *Crystal Deposition Diseases.* In *Disease-a-Month.* (Ed) HF Dowling. Year Book Medical Publishers Inc., Chicago. Page 5

McCarty, DJ and Gatter, RA (1966) *Arthritis and Rheumatism, 9,* 804

Meachim, G (1969) In *Ultrastructure of Synovial Joints in Health and Disease.* By FN Ghadially and S Roy. Butterworth, London. Page 61

Reginato, AJ, Schumacher, HR and Martinez, VA (1974) *Arthritis and Rheumatism, 17,* 977

Ruettner, JR and Spycher, MA (1968) *Pathologia et microbiologica, 31,* 14

Silberberg, R and Hasler, M (1968) *Pathologia et microbiologica, 31,* 25

Sokoloff, L (1963) *Science, 141,* 1055

Spycher, MA, Moor, H and Ruettner, JR (1969) *Zeitschrift für Zellforschung und mikroskopische Anatomie, 98,* 512

Stockwell, RA (1965) *Nature, 207,* 427

Thyberg, J and Friberg, U (1972) *Journal of Ultrastructure Research, 41,* 43

Weiss, C and Mirow, S (1972) *Journal of Bone and Joint Surgery, 54-A,* 954

Zimny, ML and Redler, I (1969) *Journal of Bone and Joint Surgery, 51-A,* 1179

12

THE INFLAMMATORY COMPONENT OF OSTEOARTHRITIS

P A Dieppe, E C Huskisson and D A Willoughby

Osteoarthritis is traditionally regarded as a non-inflammatory disease. Recently the term osteoarthrosis has been introduced emphasising the current belief that this is a degenerative condition of articular cartilage, differing fundamentally from inflammatory joint conditions such as rheumatoid arthritis. However, a number of the clinical and pathological features of osteoarthritis suggest an inflammatory component (Table I), and in this chapter it is argued that inflammation is a fundamental part of its pathogenesis. The deposition and subsequent release of crystals from articular cartilage and soft tissues is proposed as a possible mechanism for the inflammatory component.

TABLE I   Clinical and pathological features of osteoarthritis suggesting an inflammatory component

CLINICAL	PATHOLOGICAL
Often an acute polyarticular onset	Villous hypertrophy of the synovium
Variable nature of the disease	
Early morning stiffness	Patchy inflammatory cell infiltration
Inactivity stiffness	of synovium
Response to anti-inflammatory drugs	
Hot, red Heberden's nodes	Fibrous thickening of the capsule
Episodic warm effusions	
Baker's cysts, which may rupture	Synovial fluid effusions

Inflammation and Osteoarthritis

Many authors have noted that osteoarthritis is often polyarticular, the onset in many joints occuring over a short period of time, with inflammatory features being most marked in the early stages of the disease.

Following Heberden's description of nodes on the distal interphalangeal joints (Heberden, 1802), Haygarth (1805) described 34 cases of multiple arthritis associated with Heberden's nodes. Adams (1857) and Charcot (1881) also commented on the polyarticular nature of 'degenerative arthritis', and in 1926 Cecil and Archer reviewed 182 cases of osteoarthritis, finding that 145 were polyarticular and mainly affected middle aged women with Heberden's nodes ('menopausal arthritis'). Kellgren and Moore (1952) in a study of 196 cases attending a rheumatology clinic, reported only 20 monoarticular cases; they stressed the importance of an early inflammatory phase, commenting that 'each affected joint tends to pass through two stages, an initial relatively acute phase during which the joint may be warm, red and exquisitely tender, and some months later a chronic phase, characterised by bony outgrowths around the joint margins'. Stecher (1955) commented on the early tender phase in the development of Heberden's nodes, and epidemiological studies later confirmed the high incidence of polyarticular osteoarthritis and its very strong association with Heberden's nodes (Kellgren & Lawrence, 1958).

The inflammatory component of this disease may sometimes be more obvious and persistant than usual. Crain (1961) described several cases of interphalangeal osteoarthritis, a condition with marked inflammatory features, which resulted in typical Heberden's and Bouchard's nodes. Peter et al (1966) described an inflammatory subgroup of patients with osteoarthritis and bony erosions on x-ray, 'erosive osteoarthritis', and Ehrlich (1972, 1975) has described a large number of patients with 'inflammatory osteoarthritis', of whom only a small proportion later developed rheumatoid disease.

In order to investigate the frequency and possible causes of the inflammatory component of osteoarthritis, a clinicopathological study of 100 patients has been undertaken.

The Present Study

One hundred consecutive cases attending a rheumatology clinic and diagnosed clinically as having osteoarthritis entered the study. Clinical data was collected, and x-rays taken of the spine, hands, hips, knees and any other affected joints. Blood tests included haemoglobin, sedimentation rate (ESR), rheumatoid factor (SCAT), and serum calcium, phosphorus and alkaline phosphatase. In selected cases synovial fluid was aspirated and a cell count done prior to examination by polarising light microscopy and analytical electron microscopy (Crocker et al, 1977). Biopsy material was available from eight joints.

The age and sex distribution of the group was similar to those reported by Cecil and Archer (1926) and Kellgren and Moore (1952). There were 70 women and 30 men with an average age of 60.2 years (± 11.0), and the mean age at onset of symptoms was 50.5 years. Blood tests, including the ESR (mean 14.3 ± 4.1) were essentially normal and only 2% were seropositive.

The number and distribution of the affected joints is shown in Table II. The majority of cases had involvement of more than one joint site; the knees and

118

hands being most commonly affected.

Clinical signs of inflammation were common. Tender, warm swelling was often present in the knees. Of the 74 patients with knee involvement 54 (73%) had effusions, and 19 (26%) of these were warm. Baker's cysts were found in 31 (42%). Stiffness is another feature of joint diseases generally thought to be due to inflammation. Early morning stiffness and inactivity stiffness were both a feature of this group of patients (Table III).

TABLE II Joint sites involved in 100 cases of osteoarthritis.

NUMBER OF SITES INVOLVED		PRINCIPAL SITES INVOLVED	
Number	% Patients	Site	% Patients
1	18	Knees	74
2	27	Hands	62
3	20	Spine	47
4	20	Hips	32
5	10	Shoulders	17
6	2	Ankles	16
7	3	Feet	8

TABLE III Early morning stiffness and inactivity stiffness in 100 cases of osteoarthritis

TIME (Mins)	NUMBER OF PATIENTS	
	Early Morning Stiffness	Inactivity Stiffness
0	17	17
1–5	12	53
6–10	21	18
11–30	30	13
31–60	14	2
61–120	5	0
180	1	0

The x-rays were reviewed independantly by two radiologists. Definite erosions were not seen in any case; chondrocalcinosis was seen in four cases, but other abnormal areas of calcification in and around the joints was more common. The findings were otherwise those traditionally described in osteoarthritis.

Synovial fluid samples of 34 patients were examined. The findings are summarised in Table IV. Pyrophosphate crystals were identified in six cases, and nodules of hydroxyapatite were found in nine. These crystals were often intra-cellular, and a typical example of a synovial fluid white cell containing a clump of minute crystals of hydroxyapatite is shown in Figure 1. Of the eight cases in

119

TABLE IV Synovial fluid findings in 34 cases of osteoarthritis

TOTAL CELL COUNT	Range: 0.3–15.1 x 10^9 /L Mean: 3.5 ± 1.4
DIFFERENTIAL CELL COUNT	Range: 40–100% Mononuclear Mean: 79.6% Mononuclear
POLARISED LIGHT MICROSCOPY	Five cases of probable pyrophosphate crystals
ANALYTICAL ELECTRON MICROSCOPY	Six cases of pyrophosphate Nine cases of hydroxyapatite (Both crystals together in two of these cases)

whom biopsy was performed calcified nodules attached to the synovium were identified in five, and found to consist of a heavily mineralised mixture of cartilage and fibrous tissue, the mineral being identified as hydroxyapatite by infra-red spectroscopy and analytical electron microscopy. In one case a calcified area of synovium was found to contain both pyrophosphate and hydroxyapatite crystals in close proximity (Figure 2).

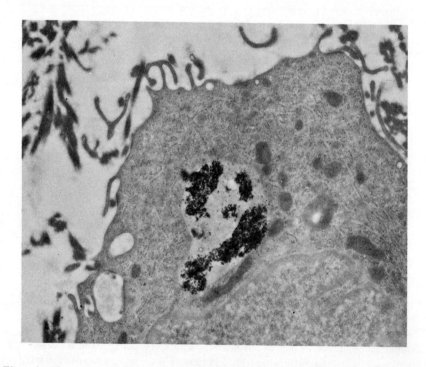

Figure 1   Phagocytic cell from the synovial fluid of a patient with osteoarthritis. Clumps of minute crystals of hydroxyapatite can be seen inside the cell (x 32,000)

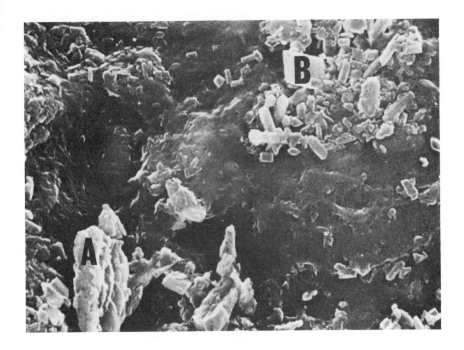

Figure 2 Scanning electron micrograph of the mineral deposit from an area of calcified synovium. Clumps of hydroxyapatite mineral (A) and calcium pyrophosphate dihydrate crystals (B) are seen in close proximity (x 10,000)

Conclusions

This study is in agreement with previous reported series which described the high incidence of polyarticular involvement and inflammatory features in osteo-arthritis. These patients, and those of Cecil and Archer (1926) and Kellgren and Moore (1952), were referred to a rheumatology clinic. A higher incidence of non-inflammatory monoarticular disease may occur in orthopaedic practice. The present series revealed a high incidence of the Galenic signs of inflammation (tenderness, heat, redness and swelling) and of stiffness. Data on the relationship between the time of onset and the occurance of inflammatory features was not available from this study, although, like others, we have seen many cases who have had an acute active onset of the disease.

Following the recent identification of hydroxyapatite crystals in synovial fluids (Dieppe et al, 1976), the incidence and type of mineral deposition in these 100 patients with osteoarthritis was investigated.

Chondrocalcinosis is known to be associated with progressive degenerative changes indistinguishable from osteoarthritis (McCarty 1975). Although only seen on the x-rays of four patients, pyrophosphate crystals were identified in six cases. However, the incidence of evidence of hydroxyapatite was far higher,

121

both radiologically and on micro-analysis of synovial fluids. These results may not indicate the true incidence of mineral deposition, since only a limited, selected number of the 100 cases could be studied. Identification of hydroxyapatite is technically difficult, and the crystals may have been missed in some negative cases. However, these results do suggest that deposition of hydroxyapatite, as described by Ali (1977), is common in osteoarthritis.

Hydroxyapatite crystals can cause inflammation (Dieppe et al, 1977), and this phenomenon is therefore a possible explanation for the inflammatory component of osteoarthritis.

References

Adams R (1857) *A treatise on rheumatic gout* , Churchill, London

Ali SY (1977) In *Perspectives in Inflammation* Eds. DA Willoughby, JP Giroud, GP Velo, MTP Press Limited

Cecil RL and Archer BH (1926) *Journal of the American Medical Association 87,* 741

Charcot JM (1881) *Clinical lectures in senile and chronic diseases,* New Sydenham Society, London

Crain DC (1961) *Journal of the American Medical Association 175,* 1049

Crocker PR, Dieppe PA, Tyler G, Chapman SK, and Willoughby DA (1977) *Journal of Pathology, 121,* 37

Dieppe PA, Huskisson EC, Crocker PR, Willoughby DA (1976) *Lancet 1,* 266

Dieppe PA (1977) In *Perspectives in Inflammation.* Eds. DA Willoughby, JP Giroud, GP Velo. MTP Press Limited

Ehrlich GE (1972) *Journal of Chronic Diseases, 25,* 317

Ehrlich GE (1975) *Journal of the American Medical Association, 232,* 157

Haygarth J (1805) *A clinical history of disease.* Cadell and Davis, London

Heberden W (1802) *Commentaries on the history and cure of diseases.* Payne, London

Kellgren JH and Lawrence JS (1958) *Annals of the Rheumatic Diseases, 17,* 388

Kellgren JH and Moore R (1952) *British Medical Journal, 1,* 181

McCarty DJ (1975) *Bulletin of Rheumatic Diseases, 25,* 804

Peter JB, Pearson CM, Marmor L (1966) *Arthritis and Rheumatism, 9,* 365

Stecher RM (1955) *Annals of the Rheumatic Diseases, 14,* 1

13

DRUG INDUCED BIOCHEMICAL CHANGES IN CARTILAGE METABOLISM

A New Concept in the Aetiopathogenesis of Osteoarthrosis

D A Kalbhen

Among the various rheumatic diseases osteoarthrosis is certainly the most frequent. In contrast to rheumatoid arthritis, which is characterised by inflammatory processes, osteoarthrosis is purely, or mainly, a degenerative disease of the articular connective tissues, and is limited to the joints. As the articular cartilage is the primary target of degenerative changes, investigation into the aetiopathogenesis of osteoarthrosis should focus on the physiological and morphological, as well as the biochemical, structural, and functional properties of joint cartilage. A good knowledge of these properties is certainly a precondition for understanding the pathological alterations and destruction of this tissue in osteoarthrosis.

Physiology of Cartilage

Normal articular cartilage consists of connective tissue cells and fibres, surrounded by a matrix, composed of proteins, polysaccharides and sulphated proteoglycans. Beneath the cartilage is subchondral bone. At the junction between the two tissues is a layer of calcified cartilage. Articular cartilage differs from other tissues in its lack of blood vessels and nerves. In the absence of a vascular system, the nutritional support and requirements of the articular cartilage as well as its intermediary metabolism are not comparable with most other tissues. As schematically demonstrated in Figure 1, nutritional substrates and metabolic end products reach or leave the connective tissue cells only by diffusion through the cartilage matrix and through the synovial fluid. From the synovial fluid substances are exchanged through the synovial membrane and the joint capsule, from where transport via blood capillaries takes place. Owing to the lack of normal oxygen supply the chondrocytes derive their energy mainly from glycolytic processes. The articular cartilage depends on perfect function of its special transport and supply system to maintain energy balance and a steady state in meta-

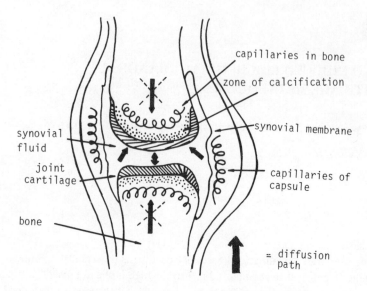

Figure 1   Schematic diagram of a joint indicating the nutritional pathways of the articular cartilage.

bolic processes. It is easy to understand, that any disturbance of this nutritional supply system will result in a reduction, or inhibition, of the metabolic requirements of the chondrocytes and may consequently result in damage to the cartilage.

Pathophysiology of Osteoarthrotic Cartilage

In osteoarthrosis the normally smooth translucent articular cartilage becomes dull and opaque with small or large areas of degeneration. Histologically there is fraying of fibres with proliferation of chondrocytes and localised necrosis. When the articular cartilage is thinned the subchondral bone becomes thickened and polished in a process called eburnation, which is generally accompanied by fibroblast proliferation and the formation of osteophytes.

The appearances of degenerative joint disease can vary depending on the site involved, but it always begins with degeneration and destruction of the cartilage.

Factors Involved

The disease is more common in the elderly but may occur at any age as a sequel to joint injury, or dysplasia through mechanical factors. However, mechanical stress does not explain all forms of osteoarthrosis. Systemic factors also seem to be important. Heberden's nodes with osteoarthrosis of the terminal interphalangeal joints are certainly not caused by mechanical stress. Some of the factors

124

TABLE I   Factors Which May Induce or Accelerate Osteoarthrosis

1. traumatic, congenital, developmental, or genetic dysplasia
2. ageing, obesity, mechanical stress
3. nutritional deficiencies, metabolic disorders
4. reduced mobility
5. drugs or environmental chemicals
6. inflammatory arthritis
7. immunological processes
8. haemophilia

involved in the development of osteoarthrosis are listed in Table I. Most factors considered in the aetiopathogenesis of osteoarthrosis will directly or indirectly disturb the nutritional requirements and metabolic activities of the articular cartilage. Examples of *indirect* inhibitory influences on cartilage nutrition are provided by animal experiments which show that immobilisation of a joint will result in osteoarthrotic degeneration (Roy, 1970; Finsterbusch & Friedmann, 1973). The experiments indicate, that the synovial fluid serves as an important carrier for nutritional substrates and metabolites, and that this carrier function is quantitatively correlated with the mobility of the joint. It seems that movements of the joint substitute in some way for a non-existing circulatory pump for synovial fluid. Following joint immobilisation the nutritional support of the cartilage tissue is inhibited and this results in a reduction or block in energy metabolism and anabolic processes in the connective tissue cells. This consequently results in slow progressive degeneration and loss of cartilage matrix.

Drug Induced Cartilage Inhibition

A more *direct* factor in the aetiopathogenesis of osteoarthrosis is drug induced inhibition of the synthetic activities of cartilage cells. This paper aims to describe the importance and relevance of this factor to osteoarthrosis.

In order to develop an experimental model of osteoarthrosis we have concentrated our efforts on pharmacological agents which induce slowly progressive degeneration in the articular cartilage of laboratory animals without provoking inflammatory reactions. A search was made for substances which would specifically interfere with anabolic processes in cartilage cells. Successful biochemical induction of osteoarthrosis in laboratory animals has been achieved in two ways:

1. As energy balance in chondrocytes is mainly dependent on glycolytic processes initial *in vitro* studies were undertaken with a potent inhibitor of glycolysis, sodium iodo-acetate. We found that this substance strongly reduced the ATP-level in cartilage as well as the synthesis of sulphated proteoglycans (Bröhr & Kalbhen, 1968; Roger & Kalbhen, 1968). Based on these results we

125

were interested to see, whether local injection of small amounts of sodium iodo-acetate into one knee joint of hens would produce similar effects. With a single or repeated dosage of 0.25 mg to 3.0 mg iodo-acetate, dissolved in 0.1 ml saline per injection, we were able to induce degeneration of the articular cartilage, which became apparent after a latent period of 2—6 weeks. This experimental osteoarthrosis was free from signs of inflammation and was progressive (Blum, 1975; Kalbhen & Blum, 1977; Kalbhen & Schiller, 1977).

TABLE II   Effect of Anti-inflammatory Drugs on Connective Tissue Metabolism

---

1. *Inhibition of Proteoglycan Synthesis by Reduction of:*
     a) Synthesis of Amino Sugars (Glucosamine and Galactosamine)
     b) Incorporation of Amino Sugars into GAG
     c) Sulphate Incorporation into GAG
     d) Incorporation of Amino Acids into Proteoglycans
2. *Inhibition of Protein Synthesis*
3. *Inhibition of Collagen Synthesis*
4. *Inhibition of Cell Proliferation*

---

2. Osteoarthrotic degeneration of articular cartilage was also induced chemi-cally with anti-inflammatory/anti-rheumatic drugs. As summarised in Table II many anti-inflammatory drugs strongly inhibit the synthesis of glycosamino-glycans, collagen and other proteins, even at therapeutic blood level concentra-tions (for reference see Trnavsky, 1974).

As there is an equilibrium of degradation and synthesis of ground substance in normal adult articular cartilage, an inhibition or reduction of synthetic pro-cesses in this tissue will result in morphological and functional changes in carti-lage. In view of the biochemical and pharmacological properties of anti-rheumatic drugs *in vitro,* we studied their effect on articular cartilage *in vivo.* After single or repeated intra-articular injections into one knee joint of hens we observed slowly progressive osteoarthrotic degeneration of the joint cartilage. The patho-logical changes, which occurred within two or three months, were similar to those in human osteoarthrosis and were identical with those induced experi-mentally by iodo-acetate.

It is interesting, and maybe characteristic for cartilage, that degeneration was not detectable earlier than four weeks, and that the degenerative changes were limited to the injected knee joint. This certainly suggests that degeneration of joint cartilage is not a systemic effect of anti-rheumatic drugs.

In the course of our experiments we investigated the osteoarthrosis-inducing effect of various anti-rheumatic drugs, as listed in Table III. Depending on dosage and drug, we found only quantitative differences in respect to time and intensity of the development of osteoarthrotic degeneration. The agent most potent in producing experimental osteoarthrosis in our laboratory animals was sodium

126

TABLE III   Experimental Osteoarthrosis Induced by Intra-articular Injection of:

Sodium Salicylate, Phenylbutazone
Oxyphenbutazone, Bumadizone
Clofezone, Flufenamic Acid
Niflumic Acid, Indomethacin,
Ibuprofen, Salicylamide
Dexamethasone—O—Phosphate
D-Penicillamine, Chloroquine Sodium Iodo-acetate

iodo-acetate. A single dose of 0.25 mg was enough to induce slowly progressive damage to the articular cartilage (Kalbhen & Schiller, 1977; Kalbhen et al,; Kalbhen & Rosenbaum, 1977; Kalbhen & Riewerts, 1977; Kalbhen & Altwein, 1977).

Experimental Results

Morphology

The macroscopic, microscopic, electron microscopic and x-ray appearances of the joints following experimental induction of osteoarthrosis are shown. As may be seen from the macroscopic pictures (Figures 2—5) the degenerative process

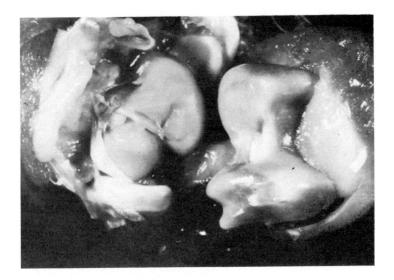

Figure 2   Macroscopic picture of an opened knee joint of a 2-year-old, healthy hen: right side — femur; left side — tibia; lower left side — fibula, (menisci and ligaments removed). The normal, thick, white and shiny cartilage is visible.

127

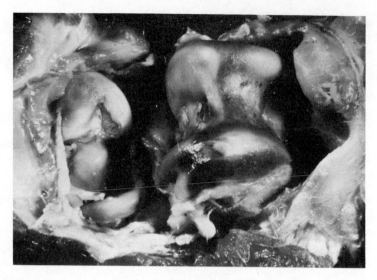

Figure 3 Cartilage surface of knee joint with early degenerative erosions and ulceration (eight weeks after intra-articular injection of phenylbutazone).

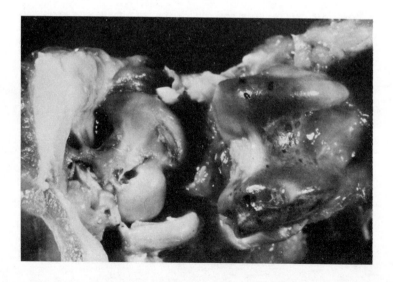

Figure 4 Very thin cartilage on femoral condyles with widespread deep ulceration and erosions; (10 weeks after intra-articular injection of sodium iodo-acetate).

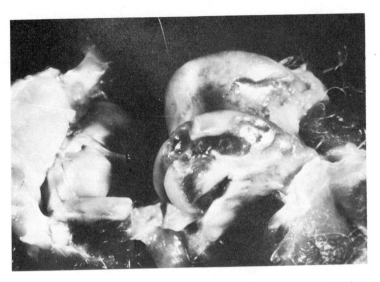

Figure 5   Severe degeneration and destruction of joint cartilage and subchondral bone; ulceration partly filled or covered with newly formed granulation tissue; (three months after a single intra-articular injection of flufenamic acid).

begins with small erosions and thinning of the cartilage and progresses to deeper ulceration and destruction, which, at a later stage may include subchondral bone.

Histology

The histological appearance of articular cartilage in the experimental osteo-arthrosis (Figures 6–9) shows the characteristic features of degenerative joint disease. The early stage of osteoarthrosis is characterised by reduced metachrom-asia and by progressive demasking of the collagen fibres. In our experiments this became visable approximately 4–6 weeks after injection of iodo-acetate or anti-rheumatic drugs (Figures 7 & 8). Within 8–12 weeks severe destruction of the cartilage surface, lamina splendens, and deep ulceration may be observed. Cluster formation of chondrocytes, newly formed granulation tissue, containing fibro-blasts, and cystic changes in subchondral bone occur. The markedly reduced metachromasia indicates inhibition of synthesis of proteoglycans by chondro-cytes.

Scanning Electron Microscopy

Using a stereoscan electron microscope the ultrastructure of the surface of articular cartilage was examined (Figures 10–12). The appearances were similar to pictures taken from human osteoarthrotic cartilage. With a magnification of

129

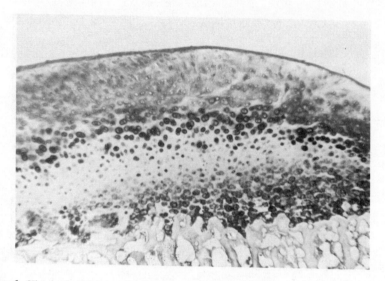

Figure 6   Histological picture of normal, healthy articular cartilage from a femoral condyle with metachromatic staining of the proteoglycan containing matrix. (Delafield's haematoxylin)

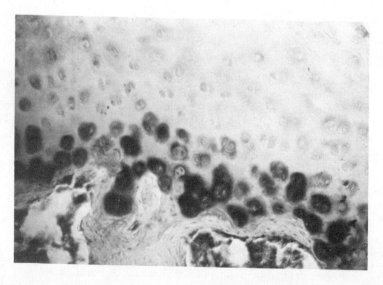

Figure 7   Reduced metachromatic staining of cartilage matrix, indicating inhibition of proteoglycan synthesis (six weeks after intra-articular injection of phenylbutazone).

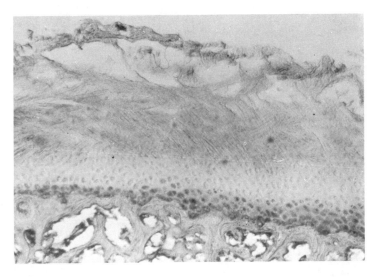

Figure 8   Destruction of cartilage surface (lamina splendens), reduced metachromasia, and demasking of collagen fibres (eight weeks after intra-articular injection of sodium iodo-acetate).

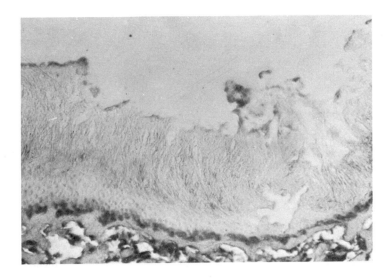

Figure 9   Ulceration and severe destruction in osteoarthrotic cartilage (10 weeks after intra-articular injection of phenylbutazone).

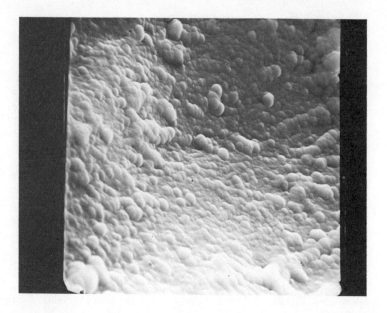

Figure 10   Stereoscan picture of intact surface of articular cartilage of the knee joint of adult healthy hen.

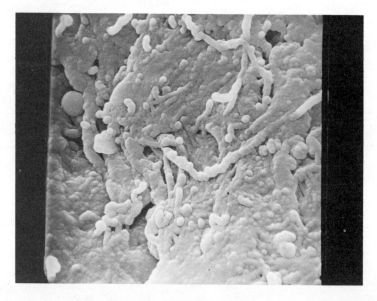

Figure 11   Stereoscan picture of cartilage surface with early depolymerisation of proteoglycans and demasking of collagen fibres.

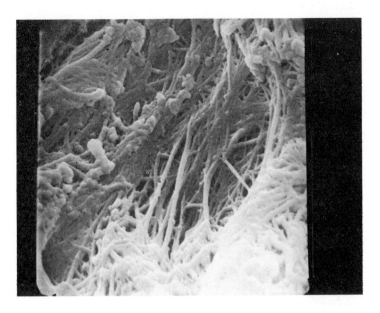

Figure 12   Stereoscan picture of cartilage surface of osteoarthrotic knee joint with severe erosions.

approximately 5000 times, normal cartilage from a femoral condyle shows a smooth and uniform surface (Figure 10).

In the early stages of osteoarthrosis depolymerisation of cartilage matrix macromolecules is associated with demasking of collagen fibres on the cartilage surface (Figure 11).

The erosions and ulceration of the articular cartilage, seen in histological slices (Figures 8 & 9) are visable as pronounced fibrillar structures (Figure 12) in stereoscan pictures of the surface of cartilage.

Biochemistry

Biochemical studies on changes in composition of the cartilage during experimental osteoarthrosis confirmed the histological findings, and have shown that the glycosaminoglycan content of cartilage is significantly reduced, depending on the intensity and duration of the degenerative process. As may be seen in Figure 13 the proteoglycan content of cartilage following iodo-acetate induced degeneration is lowered as much as 60% within 12 weeks. Similar results were obtained in experiments where phenylbutazone was used to induce experimental osteoarthrosis in laboratory animals (Figure 14). It is interesting and in keeping with our histological observations, that the DNA content of degenerative cartilage

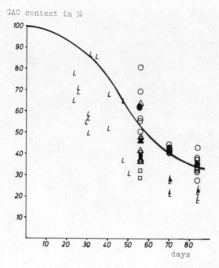

Figure 13   Reduction of proteoglycan content of cartilage with experimental osteoarthrosis induced by sodium iodo-acetate.

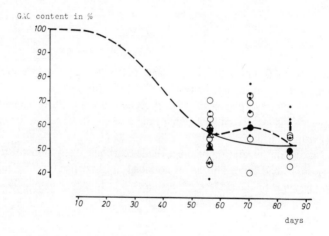

Figure 14   Reduced proteoglycan content in articular cartilage after injection of phenylbutazone.

was not significantly altered, indicating that the number of cells in cartilage tissue was not reduced.

Radiology

In order to study the progression of drug induced joint degeneration in the living

134

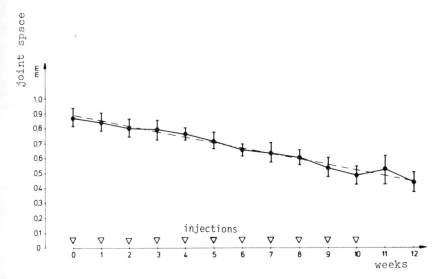

Figure 15   Decrease of joint space after weekly intra-articular injection of 5.0 mg indomethacin into the knee joint of hens (n = 8).

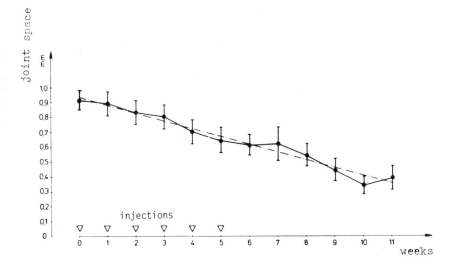

Figure 16   Decrease of joint space after intra-articular injection of niflumic acid.

animal, an x-ray method was developed using special mammography film (Kodak Definix medical) (Kalbhen & Schiller, 1977). Weekly x-ray pictures allow one to detect thinning or loss of joint cartilage by measuring the joint space. Destruction of cartilage and subchondral bone can also be studied in the living animal. The slowly progressive reduction of the joint space following repeated intra-articular injections of indomethacin and niflumic acid are shown in Figures 15 and 16.

Progressive degeneration and severe destruction involving large areas of subchondral bone were observed after only two injections of 0.5 mg sodium iodoacetate into the left knee joint of a hen (Figures 17–18). The non injected right

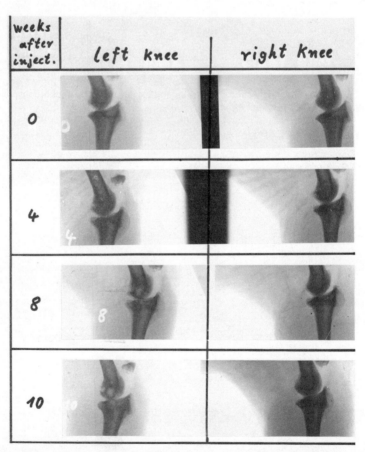

Figure 17   X-ray pictures of normal, healthy knee joints (0), and of the same joint 4, 8, 10 weeks after injection of 0.5 mg iodo-acetate into the left joint. Early signs of degeneration become visible after four weeks and cyst formation can be seen in the subchondral bone after eight and 10 weeks.

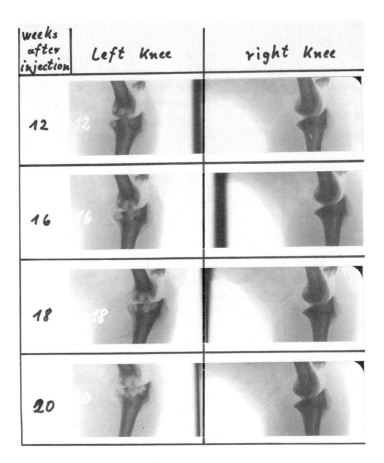

weeks after injection	Left Knee	right Knee
12		
16		
18		
20		

Figure 18   X-ray picutres of severe destruction of bone and cartilage in the left knee joint, 12, 16 18 and 20 weeks after injection of iodo-acetate. No degenerative signs in the non-injected knee joint. (Same animal as in Figure 17).

knee shows no signs of degeneration, whereas degeneration of cartilage and cystic alteration of subchondral bone were seen to be progressive four weeks after iodo-acetate injection into the left knee.

Conclusion

All the experimental data, presented in this paper, provide strong evidence that any chemically induced disturbance of the anabolic activities of cartilage cells may lead to alterations in the structural composition and functional performance of cartilage and may result in progressive degeneration. Due to the delicate and vulnerable nutritional status of the articular connective tissue any pathological inhibition of the anabolic capacity of chondrocytes will induce a self-perpetuing process of degeneration.

It is clinically well known that osteoarthrosis is a rather slowly progressive disease. As metabolic activity of cartilage cells and the turn-over rates of proteo-glycans and collagen in the cartilage matrix are very slow, there can be a long interval between the primary lesion and the first morphological evidence of cartilage degeneration. Although one must always have reservations when comparing results from animal experiments with the clinical situation of human disease, they may help us to understand physiological and pathological processes which cannot be studied in human tissues. As a result of our animal experiments, we believe that mechanical or chemical inhibitory influences on cartilage cells are potential factors in the aetiopathogenesis of osteoarthrosis.

Acknowledgments

The author wants to thank Mrs Marianne Ehses for her helpful technical assistance and Mr Manfred Lippold for photographic assistance.

Research supported by a grant from the 'Landesamt fur Forschung des Landes Nordrhein-Westfalen'.

References

Blum, U (1975) *Dissertation,* Faculty of Mathematics & Natural Sciences, University of Bonn

Bröhr, HJ and Kalbhen, DA (1968) *Archives internationales de Pharmacodynamie et de Therapie, 176,* 380

Finsterbusch, A and Friedmann, B (1973) *Clinical Orthopaedics, 92,* 305

Kalbhen, DA, Blum, U and Schiller, G (1976) *Naunyn-Schmiedebergs Archiv für Pharma-kologie,* Supplement 293, 40

Kalbhen, DA, Wentsche, B, Peil, M and Witassek, F (1976) *Paper presented at 5th Meeting, European Federation of the Connective Tissue Clubs,* Liège, Belgium

Kalbhen, DA and Altwein, T (1977) (unpublished data)

Kalbhen, DA and Blum, U (1977) *Arzneimittel-Forschung (drug research) 27,* 527

Kalbhen, DA and Riewerts, E (1977) (unpublished data)

Kalbhen, DA and Rosenbaum, C (1977) (unpublished data)

Kalbhen, DA and Schiller, G (1977) *Zeitschrift für Rheumatologie, 36,* 5

Roger, J and Kalbhen, DA (1968) *Arzneimittel-Forschung (drug research) 18,* 1512

Roy, S (1970) *Annals of the rheumatic diseases, 29,* 634

Schiller, G (1977) *Dissertation,* Faculty of Medicine, University of Bonn

Trnavsky, K (1974) In *Medicinal Chemistry, Antiinflammatory Agents, Vol 13–II,* Eds. Scherer, Whitehouse, Academic Press, London, p. 303

14

CHANGES RESEMBLING OSTEOARTHROSIS INDUCED BY THE USED CULTURE MEDIUM OF SYNOVIUM IN ORGAN CULTURE

R W Jubb and Honor B Fell

The early changes in the articular cartilage in human osteoarthrosis are loss of proteoglycan, fibrillation, loss of collagen in the matrix and proliferation of the chondrocytes to form clusters of cells (Boyle & Buchanan, 1971). Initially only the superficial part of the cartilage is affected, but as the disease progresses these alterations extend more deeply into the tissue. Precipitating factors such as trauma (Freeman, 1975), age (Collins, 1949) and genetic predisposition (Kellgren, 1961) have been suggested. Recently Glynn (1977) has postulated that the synovium may play a primary role in initiating the breakdown of cartilage in this disease. This view receives some support from the fact that in an in vitro organ culture system, synovial tissue can cause the destruction of cartilage matrix even when it is not in actual contact with the cartilage (Fell & Jubb, 1977). The experiments to be reported here, have demonstrated that degradation of cartilage matrix accompanied by some proliferation of chondrocytes occurs also in isolated cartilage grown in the used medium of synovial tissue.

Method

The object of the organ culture technique is to maintain tissues in vitro in a differentiated, functional state like that of their prototypes in the body. For our current work, the explants are cultivated in flat-bottomed vessels each containing a shallow table of stainless steel mesh on which is laid a piece of millipore membrane to serve as a substrate for the tissue. Fluid culture medium (1.5 ml of the chemically defined medium BGJ_5 with 15% normal heat-inactivated rabbit serum) is added to each vessel. The vessels are enclosed in a moist chamber and incubated in an air-tight container (for details of the method see Fell & Barratt, 1973).

The explants were taken from the metacarpo-phalangeal joints of young

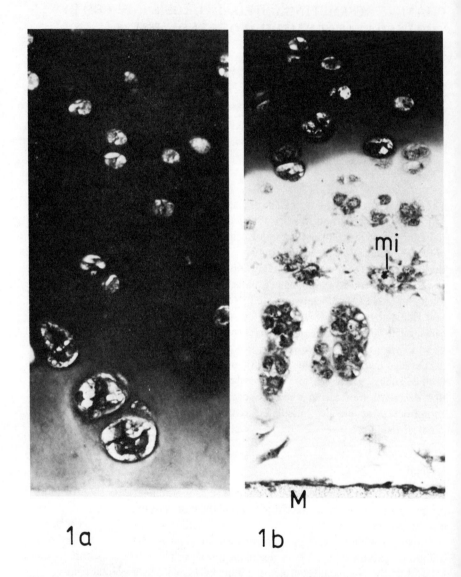

1a   1b

Figure 1   a) Section of control cartilage explant. Toluidine Blue. High power view of an
area next to the millipore membrane. Note intense staining of matrix indicating
proteoglycan. Mag. X 330.
b) Paired explant to a), cultured in synovial medium. Toluidine Blue. Note loss of
proteoglycan and proliferation of chondrocytes: M − millipore filter; mi − mitosis.
Mag. X 330.

pigs aged 5 – 9 months. In each experiment a strip of cartilage devoid of invading marrow is sliced from the distal end of each metacarpal: this is cut in half to provide paired explants, one of which is used for the test and the other for its control. Since it is technically impossible to prepare equivalent explants of the intact synovium, the synovial villi and underlying tissue are snipped from the inner surface of several sheets of joint capsule and minced with fine iridectomy scissors; the mince is pooled, centrifuged and aliquots (0.025 ml) are deposited on the millipore membrane in the culture vessels. The culture medium is changed at two-day intervals, and after the eighth and twelfth days of cultivation the used medium is collected and pooled. For the controls, medium is incubated in culture vessels without tissue. Both media are then diluted with an equal volume of fresh medium. The cartilage explants are cultured in these media for ten days after which they are fixed for histological examination.

Results

In the experiments we have done to date, the control explants underwent little histological alteration during ten days' cultivation, and in sections the matrix stained normally for sulphated proteoglycan with toluidine blue (Figure 1a) and for collagen with van Gieson's stain (Figure 2a). There was some outgrowth into the millipore membrane but otherwise little cellular change.

After cultivation in the used synovial medium, the cartilage presented a very different histological picture. Immediately above the millipore filter a broad tract of tissue was seen in which the matrix had lost its metachromasia (Figure 1b) and stained very weakly with van Gieson's stain (Figure 2b); it was obviously severely degraded. The chondrocytes had become very basophilic, sometimes showed mitosis and had formed clusters very reminiscent of those in osteoarthrotic cartilage. Sometimes the matrix had completely disappeared in certain areas and the liberated chondrocytes appeared as a mass of fibroblast-like cells.

Interpretation

The changes produced in isolated cartilage by used synovial medium are similar to those obtained when living cartilage and synovium were cultivated on the same millipore but separated from one another (Fell & Jubb, 1977): under the same conditions dead (frozen: thawed) cartilage was not affected. We concluded that this indirect effect of the synovium on the living cartilage was mediated through the chondrocytes. This view was supported by analysis of the synovial medium, which failed to reveal any active proteinases, though a collagenolytic enzyme was present in an inactive form. It is theoretically possible that the medium contained inactive enzymes which were activated

141

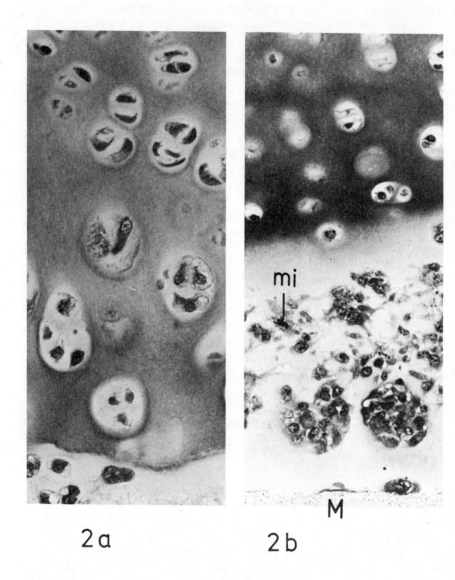

2a   2b

Figure 2   a) Same explant as in Figure 1a; van Gieson stain. Collagen intact.
Mag. x 330
b) Same explant as in Figure 1b; van Gieson stain. Loss of collagen with clusters
of chondrocytes. M—millipore, mi—mitosis.
Mag. x 330.

142

locally by the chondrocytes and then depleted the matrix, but we think it more likely that the synoviocytes liberated some substance which stimulated the cartilage cells to digest their own intercellular material. That the chondrocytes can be stimulated to act in this way was demonstrated in earlier work by Dingle et al (1975) who found that isolated pig cartilage cultivated in medium to which retinol (10 i.u./ml) had been added, lost virtually all its proteoglycan and a little of its collagen. Chondrocytes have been shown to produce proteoglycan-degrading enzymes (Sapolsky et al, 1973) and recently collagenolytic activity has also been reported (Ehrlich, 1977). Proliferation of the chondrocytes is probably a secondary effect of depletion of the matrix (Sokoloff, 1973; Millroy & Poole, 1974).

That the synoviocytes may be implicated in the pathogenesis of osteoarthrosis is suggested by the fact that sub-synovial fibrosis is a very common but hitherto unexplained feature of the disease; possibly some physiological abnormality develops in the synovium, causing it to produce some substance that induces biochemical changes in the cartilage on the one hand and sub-synovial fibrogenesis on the other.

Acknowledgments

Dame Honor B Fell is indebted to the Medical Research Council for a personal grant. The authors wish to express their thanks to the Nuffield Rheumatism Committee by whom the expenses of the research was defrayed and to Professor RRA Coombs, FRS for providing laboratory accommodation, also to Mr R Green for preparing the plates.

References

Boyle JA, Buchanan WW, (1971) *Clinical Rheumatology,* Blackwell Scientific Publications, Oxford, p. 17

Collins DH (1949) *The Pathology of articular and spinal diseases, pp 74–115* Arnold, London

Dingle JT, Horsfield P, Fell Honor B, Barratt MEJ, (1975) *Annals of the Rheumatic Diseases, 34,* 303

Ehrlich MG, Mankin HJ, Jones H, Wright R, Crispen C, Vigliani G, (1977) *The Journal of Clinical Investigation, 59,* 226

Fell HB, Barratt MEJ, (1973) *International Archives of Allergy and Applied Immunology, 44,* 441

Fell HB, Jubb RW, (1977) *Arthritis and Rheumatism, 20,* 1359

Freeman MAR, (1975) *Annals of the Rheumatic Diseases, 34 suppl.* p.120

Glynn LE, (1977) *Lancet 1,* 574

Kellgren JH, (1961) *British Medical Journal, 2,* 1

Millroy SJ, Poole AR, (1974) *Annals of the Rheumatic Diseases, 33,* 500

Sapolsky AI, Altman RD, Howell DS, (1973) *Federation Proceedings, 32,* 1489

Sokoloff L, (1973) *Normal and Osteoarthritic Articular Cartilage.* Eds. SY Ali, MW Elves, DH Leaback, Kingswood Press, p. 113

15

IDENTIFICATION OF IMMUNOGLOBULINS AND COMPLEMENT COMPONENTS IN ARTICULAR COLLAGENOUS TISSUES OF PATIENTS WITH IDIOPATHIC OSTEOARTHROSIS

T D V Cooke, E L Bennett and O Ohno

The aetiology of osteoarthrosis is unclear. Some consider the pathological manifestations as being the final common pathway of multiple causes (Solomon, 1976, Lee et al, 1974). Others suspect biochemical and/or mechanical mechanisms as the cause of cartilage disease, potentially triggered by many non-specific agents (Meachim & Collins, 1965; Bollet, 1969; Mankin et al, 1971; Radin et al, 1970; Todd et al, 1972).

The pathogenesis of hip disease has been subject to much discussion (Solomon, 1976; Plewes, 1940; Lloyd-Roberts, 1955; Harmon, 1942; Harrison et al, 1953) and experimental study (Mankin et al, 1971; Radin et al, 1970) but few reports detail clinical or radiologic manifestations of other diseased joints in these patients.

Significant inflammatory synovitis and an aggressive and/or destructive course of osteoarthrosis have been identified in association with crystal deposition in pseudogout (Gerster et al, 1975; Menkes et al, 1976), and more recently suggested in association with hydroxyapatite crystal disease (Schumacher, 1977; Dieppe et al, 1976).

Studies have either confirmed (Kellgren & Moore, 1952; Kellgren et al, 1963; Roh et al, 1973) or refuted (Stecher, 1961, 1965; Yazici et al, 1975) the relationship between the presence of Heberden's nodes and large weight-bearing joint and/or spine involvement. With regard to hand presentation however, the interrelationships and overlaps between inflammatory osteoarthrosis and rheumatoid arthritis (RA) were detailed with great clarity by Ehrlich (1972b). He noted the remarkable symmetry of involvement and the extent of disease in the spine and large joints (Ehrlich, 1972a & b).

The majority of osteoarthrosic patients presenting to our treatment centre have had hip or knee disease without obvious predisposing factors. For study purposes we have termed these cases 'idiopathic'.

Many others present with definite evidence of a specific mechanism such as dysplasia, previous trauma or neurological disease as inciting agents. These have been designated as 'secondary'. Excluded are patients with inflammatory arthritis that have developed secondary osteoarthrosic manifestations.

In an attempt to define the prevalence of immunoglobulins (Ig) and complement components (β1c) in articular cartilage biopsies of joints with various arthritides, as controls for rheumatoid arthritis, we noted a significant prevalence of positive staining reactions in cases of osteoarthrosis (Cooke et al, 1975a; Cooke & Bennett, 1976). The presence of specific staining for at least two Igs and β1c in an identical location were the criteria for complex deposition (Cooke et al, 1975(b)).

This chapter reviews data obtained from over 100 cases of osteoarthrosis that comprise both secondary and idiopathic groups.

Our aim in current and future studies is to clarify the involvement of local immune mechanisms that involve cartilage in idiopathic osteoarthrosis and to compare this to what is known in rheumatoid arthritis. We hope to gain information that will aid in the differentiation of primary disease states.

Materials and Methods

Patient Study Protocols

This work documents an extension of a prospective cartilage biopsy study that has been previously described (Cooke et al, 1975a; Cooke & Bennett, 1976). A variety of patients, requiring surgical reconstruction for various arthropathies were clinically documented and agreed to laboratory investigations that included haematology, sedimentation rate, autoantibody levels, (rheumatoid factors by latex fixation and sensitised sheep cell tests, and antinuclear antibody activity), SMA$_{12}$, serum protein electrophoresis, immunoglobulin and complement levels. Radiographs of the involved joints were also obtained.

The major groups studied to this time include: Group 1 — non-arthritic 29, Group II — secondary osteoarthrosic 32, Group III — idiopathic osteoarthrosic 85, and Group IV — classical R.A. 97. The presentation centres on the analysis of the 117 osteoarthrosic cases. Sixty three biopsied cases designated idopathic (Group III) have had their documentation and radiographs re-evaluated.

Immunofluorescent Reagents

Monospecific sheep antisera against human IgG, IgM, IgA and β1c obtained from Dr J. Bienenstock (Professor of Medicine, Host Resistence Programme, McMaster University Medical Centre, Hamilton, Ontario, Canada), have been already characterised (Cooke et al, 1975b). They were conjugated with fluorescein isothiocyanate by standard techniques (Weir, 1967).

145

Articular Tissue Biopsies

At surgery, articular surface slices of hyaline cartilage, menisci and ligaments were obtained from resected tissues. After washing in phosphate buffered saline (PBS) they were immersed vertically in freezing medium (Tissue-Tek OCT Compound Ames T.M.Co.) within plastic containers, snap frozen in liquid nitrogen and stored at -70°C.

Specimen Preparation and Immunofluorescent Staining

Thin sections that included the articular surface were obtained as previously described and after washing were stained with monospecific fluoresceinated antisera against each Ig and β1c using suitable 'blocking' controls (Cooke et al, 1975a). After extensive washing in PBS they were read in a dry dark field using a Zeiss Universal microscope with fluorescein excitation by ultraviolet light from an Osram Mercury Bulb (HBO 200), exciting filters BG 38 and two FITC 495s with number 53 barrier filters. Photomicrographs were taken on Kodak Tri-X film (Eastman Kodak).

Results

Incidence of Complex Deposition in Major Study Groups

A total of 77 biopsies have been added to the study groups. They include nine non-arthritics, seven secondary osteoarthrosic, 25 idiopathic osteoarthrosic and 21 classical RA cases. The immunofluorescent staining reactions for complexes in each group are shown in Table I. Only one of 29 non-arthritic cases (Group I) has had positive findings. This hyaline cartilage biopsy was obtained from a recent elbow fracture and had positive staining on the surfaces that were otherwise normal.

TABLE I   The Immunofluorescence Staining Reactions in Major Groups Studied

Group	Description	Biopsies studied	Per cent positive
I	Non-arthritic	29	3
II	Secondary osteoarthrosis	32	16
III	Idiopathic osteoarthrosis	89	51
IV	Classical rheumatoid	95	92

As before, classical RA cases (Group IV) have had a greater than 92% incidence of positive findings. Staining patterns were often intense and extensive and included menisci, ligaments and diseased tendons (Cooke et al, 1975b).

The overall incidence of positive reactions in cases classed as secondary osteoarthrosis (Group II) was 16% . Their aetiological breakdown is shown in Table II.

146

TABLE II Immunofluorescence Staining Reactions of Hyaline Articular Cartilage in Secondary Osteoarthrosis* (Group II)

Secondary Osteoarthrosis	Number biopsied	Number positive	Per cent positive
Trauma	21	4	19
Dysplasia	9	1	11
Neurogenic	2	0	0
Total	32	5	16

* Subsequent re-evaluation of the records and radiographs in 63 Group III cases identified eight, all with negative biopsies, as probably secondary to dysplasia (6), osteonecrosis (1) and trauma (1). When included in the above the percentage of positive reactions is reduced to 13.

Trauma accounted for 21 with four positive whereas one of nine dysplastics and none of neurogenic cases were positive (the findings in a subsequent re-evaluation of Group III cases suggest the addition of eight cases, all with negative biopsies, as secondary to dysplasia (6), osteonecrosis (1) and old trauma (1). These reduce the overall incidence of positives to <14% (see Table VIII)).

Fifty-one percent of the 85 idiopathic osteoarthrosic cases had positive staining reactions as shown in Table III. The prevalence varied somewhat in previous studies (Cooke et al, 1975b; Cooke & Bennett, 1976) but the larger number of cases now collected clarify these data (Table IV) and indicate a statistically significant difference in prevalence in both secondary disease (p<.005), and non-arthritics (p< .001).

TABLE III Immunofluorescent Staining Reactions of Hyaline Cartilage Biopsies in Idiopathic Osteoarthrosis

Number patients	Number biopsies	Number positive	Per cent positive
85*	89	45	51

* Four patients had two joints biopsied.

TABLE IV Statistical Analysis of the Incidence of Complex Deposition in Cartilage Biopsies of Idiopathic Osteoarthrosis Compared to Secondary and Non-Arthritic Cases

Arthritic Groups	Total number	Number positive	Number positive	p Value III vs I and II
I Non-arthritic	29	1	3	< .001
II Secondary osteoarthrosis	32	5	16	< .005
III Idiopathic osteoarthrosis	89	45	51	- - -

Immunofluorescent Staining Patterns in Positive Osteoarthrosic and RA Cases

The occurrence of complement fixing immune complexes is suggested when Igs and β_{1c} are identified at an identical location. In idiopathic osteroarthrosis the Igs identified most often were IgA and IgG. The former was usually the more intense, well localised to surfaces and included cell staining. This pattern contrasted with a lack of IgA cell staining in RA. Meniscal and ligament tissue surfaces stained for IgA and usually IgG, whereas in RA, staining was more intense, consistent and throughout the tissue following the collagen fibre architecture.

In osteoarthrosis IgG staining was seen diffusely in the cartilage matrix as deep as 0.3 mm in low concentration. It was sometimes absent. In RA the staining, in contrast, was nearly always strong and most consistently IgG in a granular, intense pattern at the surface. An 'RA pattern' for IgG was occasionally found in osteoarthrosis. IgM staining was seldom observed and when present was patchy and low in intensity.

In osteoarthrosis a low to medium intensity fluorescence for β_{1c} occurred at the surfaces associated with weak staining of the cells. In RA, stronger surface staining, not involving the cells was commonly found.

Comparison of Demographic and Laboratory Features in Osteoarthrosis

A comparison of demographic data in secondary and idiopathic groups is shown in Table V. Similar age means but an opposite sex distribution was found, with

TABLE V Demographic Features in Osteoarthrosis

Group	Number biopsies	Mean age (years)	Sex Ratio F	M	Disease duration (years)
II Secondary	32	64	1	1.4	17
III Idiopathic	89	69	2.2	1	9

TABLE VI Laboratory Parameters in Osteoarthrosis

Group	Number biopsies	ESR* mm/hr	Number positive RF☆	Number positive ANA¶	Histological grade†	Per cent complex positive
II Secondary	32	34	0 of 10	0 of 10	1	16
III Idiopathic	89	36	5 of 57	14 of 55	2.1	51

*   ESR Erythrocyte Sedimentation Rate
☆   RF Positivity of either slide latex or sensitised sheep cell at a titre of >1 in 16
¶   ANA Positivity − antinuclear positivity at a dilution of >1 in 20
†   Based on lymphocyte and plasma cell infiltration graded 0−6

a 2 to 1 female to male ratio in idiopathic arthritis. Another difference was the almost two fold greater disease duration in secondary cases.

There was no difference in mean sedimentation rates (Table VI). The idiopathic group had a higher incidence of seropositivity for rheumatoid and antinuclear factor activity, twice the grade levels for synovial infiltration with lymphocytes and plasma cells and a nearly four fold prevalence of complex deposition when compared with secondary group II cases.

Comparison of Data in Complex Positive and Negative Cases of Idiopathic Arthritis

When the positively and negatively reacting cases in the idiopathic group were compared few differences were found. These are shown in Table VII. They include a slightly greater mean age, disease duration and histological grades in

TABLE VII Data Comparison in Complex Positive and Negative Biopsied Cases of Idiopathic Osteoarthrosis

	Whole group means	Complex	
		Negative	Positive
Age	69	67	73
Duration years	9.1	7	11
Synovial histologic grade	2.1	1.9	2.3
Sex ratio Female : Male	2 : 1	NS	
Sedimentation rate	36	NS	
RF per cent positive	11	NS	
ANA per cent positive	22	NS	

NS = No significant difference

positive staining cases. No obvious differences were seen in sex ratios, sedimentation rates, and autoantibody activities as they related to staining reaction.

Re-evaluation of Documentation and Radiographs in Biopsied Cases of Idiopathic Osteoarthrosis

Since rheumatoid-like cases might be intermixed within the degenerative group, and provide an abnormally high incidence of positivity, we re-evaluated the documentation and radiographs in 63 biopsied cases grouped as idiopathic osteoarthrosis. Eleven of these were reclassified as shown in Table VIII. Only 3 were polyarthritic, 2 with rheumatoid-like and one with an asymmetrical psoriatic-like pattern. All had positive biopsies. Eight negatively staining cases had strong

149

TABLE VIII Diagnostic Group of Re-evaluated Biopsied Cases in Idiopathic
Osteoarthrosis (Group III)

Number re-evaluated	63	(34)
Number remaining Group III	52	(31)
Number reclassified	11	(03)
Inflammatory polyarthritis*	03	(03)
Secondary dysplasia – Hip	02	(0)
dysplasia – Knee†	04	(0)
osteonecrosis – Knee	01	(0)
old trauma – Knee	01	(0)

( )   Numbers in parentheses are cases with positive immunofluorescent staining for
complexes

*   Two cases with RA distribution, one case – asymmetrical psoriatic-like pattern

†   Developmental overgrowth of medial femoral and lateral tibial condyles providing
an oblique joint line and gross subluxation

evidence of a joint abnormality likely to induce their arthritis. In two hips this
was dysplasia of a classical acetabular form (Wiberg, 1939) and in four knees
the dysplasia was the development of an oblique joint line, due to relative overgrowth of medial femoral and lateral tibial condyles, and subsequent gross subluxation (Kettelkamp et al, 1975; Surin et al, 1975). One knee was associated
with femoral osteonecrosis and another with old trauma. When these eight
cases are added to Group II data the overall incidence of positive findings falls
from 16 to about 13% (5 of 40).

TABLE IX The Relationship of Cartilage Staining Reactions to the Site of Biopsy and
Sex of Re-evaluated Patients with Idiopathic Osteoarthritis (Group III)

Site	Number biopsied	Number positive	Sex ratio F	M
Knee	16	8	6.5	1
Feet	2	2	–	
Hips	34	23	1	1
Totals	52	31	2 :	1

The review of the remaining 52 cases seen in Table IX, shows nearly equal
numbers of positive and negative biopsies from knees, with a high female preponderance in both subgroups. Hip biopsies were twice as common as knees
with positive reactions in two-thirds. The sex ratio in positive hips was 2.1
female to male, while, negatively staining biopsies were most often male. The

two joints from the feet examined were both positive. The majority of cases had bilateral involvement and collectively the review yielded an overall 63% of positive reactions, with a two to one female to male ratio.

Relationship of Biopsy Sites to Staining Reactions in Osteoarthrosis

It was possible that the high incidence of positive reactions in hip biopsies might be due to the biopsied joint being covered with blood at surgery. The staining reactions in hips and knees were therefore compared in Groups II and III and are shown in Table X. Fourteen per cent of hips from secondary arthritics were

TABLE X Comparison of Cartilage Staining Reactions of Hip and Knee Biopsies in Osteoarthrosis*

Group	HIP			KNEE		
	Number	Number positive	Per cent positive	Number	Number positive	Per cent positive
II Secondary osteoarthrosis	22	3	14	18	0	0
III Idiopathic osteoarthrosis	34	23	68	16	8	50

*   Data presented is subsequent to radiological review

positive compared to nearly 70% in idiopathic cases in spite of similar surgical circumstances. None of the secondary knee cases were positively compared to half of the idiopathic group; both had been biopsied under tourniquet.

Discussion

Our previous information (Cooke et al, 1975a; Cooke & Bennett, 1976) on the incidence of positive immunofluorescent staining reactions in osteoarthrosis was limited by lack of representative numbers in the major subgroups. The data presented indicate positive findings in at least 50% of idiopathic cases and an incidence of no more than 15% in secondary arthritis. The incidence of positive findings in Group III is highly significantly more than in non-arthritics and less than in classical RA ($p < .001$ in both instances).

As our experience with immunofluorescent staining of collagenous tissues grows so subtle differences in staining between positive cases of osteoarthrosis and RA biopsies are suggested. These impressions are summarised in Table XI. Preliminary unpublished data (Ohno & Cooke, 1977) using immuno-electron-microscopic techniques have indicated dense concentrations of IgG aggregated in a highly structured form in RA collagenous surfaces. Even more preliminary is the data is osteoarthrosis which also suggests a form of Ig deposition in some

151

TABLE XI Immunofluorescent Staining Patterns in Osteoarthrosis and RA

Antisera against	Osteoarthrosis	Rheumatoid Arthritis
IgA	Concentrated, surface localised, consistent, ++ cell staining	Linear, medium intensity, consistent ± granular, – cell staining
IgG	Diffuse, low intensity up to 0.3 mm deep, inconsistent, – cell staining. (Occasionally like RA)	Intense, constant, granular, less than 0.2mm deep, ± cell staining
IgM	Inconstant, patchy, low intensity, + faint cell staining	Usually present, patchy, variable intensity, – cell staining
β_{1c}	Follows IgA pattern, low/ medium intensity + cell staining	Follows IgG pattern, often intense and granular, – cell staining

cases, but differing in size, pattern and concentration to that in RA. The findings are at variance to the ultrastructural staining patterns for IgG reported by Ishikawa et al (1975). Our information lends support to the suggestion that the positive immunofluorescent reactions in idiopathic osteoarthrosis are due to immune complex deposition, but probably of a different nature and pattern to that in RA.

A lack of staining reactions is a significant feature of Group III cases in both hip and knee biopsies and suggests that complex deposition, if it occurs, may come and go, or occur early or late in the disease. Our information is insufficient to clarify this question as yet.

The differences between demographic and laboratory features of the secondary and idiopathic groups are probably meaningful. Thus, the age means and sedimentation rate values are similar, yet a significant number of Group III have autoantibody reactivity, a markedly different sex ratio, with female preponderance of two to one, and shorter disease duration. Further, Group III synovial biopsies had a more than two fold higher grade for lymphocyte and plasma cell infiltration, and this was associated with a markedly different incidence of positive cartilage reactivity (p < .005). These differences lend support to their clinical designation as at *least* two distinct groups.

Within Group III few features were found that correlated for or against complex deposition. Of interest was the increased histological grading, greater mean age and disease duration. Two-thirds of the re-evaluated hips, half of the knee cases and both of two feet had positive biopsies. These data are as yet without other correlations, and do not bear much emphasis except to state that false positives due to blood on the tissue cannot account for the findings.

Synovial infiltrates of lymphocytes and plasma cells suggest local immune reactivity. This appears to relate to the prevalence of immune complex deposition

152

in idiopathic osteoarthrosis and suggests a direct relationship. Its involvement in mechanisms of cartilage disease is not yet clear.

Superimposed rheumatoid disease on a background of osteoarthrosis has been seen but in the format of this study such patients would be grouped as rheumatoid or other inflammatory polyarthritis. Our impression is that the incidence of such an occurrence in our cases is low, and of the order reported for inflammatory osteoarthritis (Ehrlich, 1972b) and cannot account for the findings observed.

It is our clinical impression that many of these cases have a polyarticular, symmetrically disposed pattern of largely asymptomatic arthritis. The preliminary results of clinical and radiological prospective assessment with laboratory and biopsy correlation support this view (Bennett & Cooke, 1977). A suitable control population is a necessity.

These data suggest that idiopathic osteoarthrosis presenting with knee and/or hip disease may have a polyarticular disease pattern (Kellgren & Moore, 1952) with a 2 : 1 female to male ratio, evidence for greater than normal serum autoantibody reactivity and varying grades of chronic synovitis that relate positively to cartilage staining for immunoglobulins and complement. The fluorescence patterns suggest a distinct form of complex deposition in these tissues. The data gathered to this time are consistent with the idea that a primary arthritic disease process involving local immune mechanisms on a temporal basis is responsible for the cartilage destruction.

Acknowledgments

The authors are particularly grateful to Dr John Wyllie, Department of Pathology, Queen's University, who has aided in the histological assessment of synovium, and the surgeons and physicians involved in the Rheumatic Disease Unit for their support. They wish also to acknowledge the expert technical assistance of Mrs L Wright, Mr E Winker and the diligent secretarial work of Miss J Pringle and Mrs J Cooke.

References

Bennett, E and Cooke, TDV (1977) *Unpublished observations*
Bollet, AJ (1969) *Arthritis and Rheumatism, 12,* 152
Cooke, TDV and Bennett, EL (1976) *Proceedings of the 22nd Annual Orthopaedic Research Society, 43,* 45
Cooke, TDV, Hurd, ER, Jasin, HE, Bienenstock, J and Ziff, M (1975b) *Arthritis and Rheumatism, 18,* 541
Cooke, TDV, Richer, S, Hurd, E and Jasin, HE (1975a) *Annals of the New York Academy of Sciencies, 256,* 10
Dieppe, PA, Huskisson, EC, Crocker, P and Willoughby, DA (1976) *Lancet, i,* 266
Ehrlich, GE (1972a) *Journal of Chronic Diseases, 25,* 317
Ehrlich, GE (1972b) *Journal of Chronic Diseases, 25,* 635

Gerster, JC, Vischer, TL, Boussina, I and Fallet, GH (1975) *British Medical Journal, 4,* 684

Harmon, PH (1942) *Pennsylvania Medical Journal, 45,* 948

Harrison, MHM, Schajawicz, F and Trueta, J (1953) *Journal of Bone and Joint Surgery, 35B,* 598

Ishikawa, H, Smiley, JD and Ziff, M (1975) *Arthritis and Rheumatism, 18,* 563

Kellgren, JH and Moore, R (1952) *British Medical Journal, 1,* 181

Kellgren, JH, Lawrence, JS and Bier, F (1963) *Annals of the Rheumatic Diseases, 22,* 237

Kettelkamp, DB, Leach, RE and Nasca, R (1975) *Clinical Orthopaedics and Related Research, 106,* 232

Lee, P, Rooney, PJ, Sturrock, RD, Kennedy, AC and Dick, WC (1974) *Seminars in Arthritis and Rheumatism, 3,* 189

Lloyd-Roberts, GC (1955) *Journal of Bone and Joint Surgery, 37B,* 8

Mankin, HJ, Dorfman, H, Lippiello, L and Sarins, A (1971) *Journal of Bone and Joint Surgery, 53A,* 523

Meachim, G and Collins, DH (1965) *Annals of Rheumatic Diseases, 21,* 45

Menkes, CJ, Simon, F, Delrieu, F, Forest, M and Delbarre, F (1976) *Arthritis and Rheumatism, 19,* 329

Ohno, O and Cooke, TDV (1977) *Unpublished observations*

Plewes, LW (1940) *British Journal of Surgery, 27,* 682

Radin, EL, Paul, IL and Tolkoff, MJ (1970) *Arthritis and Rheumatism, 13,* 400

Roh, YS, Dequeker, J and Mulier, JC (1973) *Clinical Orthopaedics and Related Research, 90,* 90

Schumacher, HR, Somlyo, AP, Tse, RL and Maureur, K (1977) *Annals of Internal Medicine, 87,* 411

Solomon, L (1976) *Journal of Bone and Joint Surgery, 58B,* 176

Stecher, RM (1961) *Geriatrics, 16,* 167

Stecher, RM (1965) *Archives of Physical Medicine and Rehabilitation, 46,* 178

Surin, V, Markhede, G and Sundholm, K (1975) *Acta Orthopaedica Scandinavica, 46,* 996

Todd, RC, Freeman, MAR and Price, CJ (1972) *Journal of Bone and Joint Surgery, 54B,* 723

Weir, DM (1967) *Handbook of Experimental Immunology,* Blackwell Scientific, Oxford, p. 579

Wiberg, G (1939) *Acta Chirurgica Scandinavica Suppt. 58,* 155

Yazici, H, Saville, PD, Salvati, EA, Bohne, WHO and Wilson, PD Jr. (1975) *Journal of the American Medical Association, 231,* 1256

16

THE GEOGRAPHY OF OSTEOARTHROSIS

J S Lawrence and M Sebo

In a comparison of degenerative joint disease in population samples in Northern Europe osteoarthrosis was least common in the most northerly males, only 1% having x-ray changes in more than half the joints in Heinola at 61°N compared with 6% in Leigh at 53°N (Lawrence et al, 1963). Blumberg and his colleagues (1961) found a similarly low prevalence in Alaska at 70°N when compared with Washington. It is clear that if a convincing proof of a relationship between latitude and the prevalence of degenerative joint disease is to be obtained a wider variation of latitude must be studied.

With this in mind a series of x-rays from population samples varying in latitude from 54°North to 26°South has been graded for osteoarthrosis (Table I). The methods of sampling and completion rate in the earlier surveys have already been described (Bennett & Wood, 1968).

Of the newer studies the Azmoos survey was an area survey based on the village of Azmoos in the Canton of St. Galen in Switzerland. All ages were included. The men in this population are largely farmers. Some of the women work in a textile mill (Zinn, 1970).

The surveys in Nigeria and Liberia were based on the villages of Igbo-Ora and Isheri and the rubber plantation of Cavalla. It was designed as an age-stratified sample but accurate stratification proved impossible (Muller, 1970).

The Phokeng survey comprised the total population of the village of Phokeng, 60 miles west of Pretoria in the Transvaal. The population is of negro stock and the main occupation is farming (Beighton et al, 1975). The Soweto survey was based on the negro township of Orlando East in Johannesburg. Fifteen blocks of houses were selected at random and all persons of pure negro stock living in these blocks were included (Solomon et al, 1975).

Altogether there were 17 population samples of which six were urban and eleven rural. Nine of the populations were Caucasians four negro and four Amerindian. The present study is concerned only with those aged 35 and over.

155

TABLE I   Routine X-rays in Surveys Used In This Study

Site	Latitude	Longitude	Age group x-rayed routinely					
			Hands	Cervical spine	Lumbar spine	Pelvis	Knees	Feet
Queen Charlotte Islands	54°N	132°W	15+	15+	–	M 15+	–	15+
Wensleydale	54°N	2°W	15+	15+	35+	55+	35+	15+
Leigh	53°N	2°W	15+	15+	35+	55+	35+	15+
Rhondda	51°N	3°W	35–64	35–64	–	–	–	35–64
Glamorgan	51°N	3°W	55–64	55–64	55–64	–	–	55–64
Watford	51°N	0°W	15+	15+	35+	M 15+ F 45+	35+	15+
Oberhörlen (1963)	50°N	8°E	15+	15+	–	–	–	15+
Oberhörlen (1968)	°		15+	15+	–	M 15+ F 45+	–	15+
Montana	48°N	113°W	30+	30+	–	M 30+ F 45+	–	30+
Piéstany	48°N	18°E	35+	35+	–	35+	35+	35+
Azmoos	47°N	9°E	5+	–	–	5+	5+	5+
Tecumseh	42°N	84°W	35+	35+	–	–	–	–
New Haven	41°N	73°W	15+	–	–	–	–	15+
Arizona	33°N	112°W	30+	30+	–	M 30+ F 45+	–	30+
Jamaica	18°N	76°W	35–64	35–64	35–64	M 35–64 F 45–64	35–64	35–64
Nigeria	4°N	3°E	25+	25+	–	M 25+ F 45+	–	25+
Liberia	4°N	3°E	25+	25+	–	M 25+ F 45+	–	25+
Phokeng	26°S	27°E	5+	–	–	–	–	5+
Soweto	26°S	28°E	5+	–	–	–	–	5+

156

The x-rays taken as a routine on all respondents are shown in Table I. Only the hands were x-rayed in all surveys but the feet were included in all except the Tecumseh survey and the neck was omitted only in the Azmoos, New Haven and South African surveys. The pelvis was x-rayed in 12 of the 17 surveys and the knees in six. In Jamaica and the Rhondda only those aged 35–64 were included. Only x-rays of persons aged 35 and over from the Tecumseh survey were read for the purpose of this study.

All x-rays were read by one observer. The x-rays from the various surveys were intermingled and so far as possible the observer was kept in ignorance of the population survey from which each x-ray had come. Some of the surveys were read more than once, notably those from Leigh, Wensleydale, Watford and Jamaica, so that comparison could be made with later surveys from other countries. In this way it was possible to exclude intra-observer variation as a cause of any 'geographical' differences in prevalence which might be observed.

The x-rays were graded for osteoarthrosis in accordance with the Atlas of Standard Radiographs of Arthritis (1963 & Lawrence, 1977).

Results

Number of Joint Groups with Osteoarthrosis (O.A.)

The number of joint groups has been used as in previous publications to give a

TABLE II Number of Joint Groups with Grade 2–4 Osteoarthrosis in Hands, Feet and Neck in Different Population Samples (1963–5 Readings)

Site and age		Males				Females			
	Total x-rayed	Unweighted mean per cent			Total x-rayed	Unweighted mean per cent			
		1+	3+	5+		1+	3+	5+	
Queen Charlotte Islands 35+	119	60	23	4	93	51	12†	3	
Wensleydale 35+	293	58	16NS	3	349	67	23	6	
Leigh 35+	530	67	20	5	600	73¶	30	8	
Watford 35+	118	62	23	10	135	63	22	10NS	
Oberhörlen (1963) 35+	112	57	8	2	147	50†	18	2	
Montana 35+	521	55	16*	3	410	53	15	2	
Tecumseh 35+	198	42	16	3	201	50‡	17	6	
Arizona 35+	417	67	31	11	396	53	15	3	
Jamaica 35–64	259	44	6*	0.8	267	53	10	1	
All surveys 35+	2567	60	20	5	2598	60	22	6	
35–64	2082	51	10	1	2103	50	9	1	

*P ≈.05   † .05 >P> .01   ‡ P < .01   ¶ P < .005

157

numerical assessment of the amount of O.A.; in particular of generalised osteoarthrosis in the population. A joint group is defined for this purpose as all those joints having the same appelation, i.e. all the distal interphalangeal joints of the fingers.

The x-rays read in 1963—5 are considered in Table II and are based on the hands, feet and neck. The data are based on unweighted means of the age groups 35—44, 45—54 and 55—64.

In the group as a whole there was little difference between the sexes, 60% of males and 60% of females aged 35 or over having osteoarthrosis in one joint or other. Three plus joint groups were affected in 20% of men and 22% of women and five plus joint groups in 5% and 6% respectively. There were however in some populations quite marked sex differences in the amount of generalised osteoarthrosis. For example in Leigh where there was more in females (P ≈.0002) and also in Wensleydale (P ≈ .03) and Oberhörlen (P ≈ .02). In the Haida Indians in the Queen Charlotte Islands on the other hand the prevalence of generalised osteoarthrosis was greater in males (P ≈ .03) as it was in the Pima Indains in Arizona (P < .0001).

The prevalence of osteoarthrosis was unrelated to latitude or longitude. The greatest prevalence (1+ joint groups) was observed in Leigh, Lancashire and the lowest in the population of Tecumseh in Michigan; but the Blackfeet Indians in Montana, USA also had a low prevalence. Comparing each population with the mean for all populations and using all ages from 35 onwards, the highest prevalence in males was in Arizona where 11% had osteoarthrosis in five or more joint groups compared with 5% for all males (P < .0001). The males in Watford also had more than the expected amount (P ≈ .02). Somewhat low prevalences at the three plus level were found in males in Montana and Jamaica (P ≈ .05) and at the one plus level in Tecumseh.

Of the females, those in Leigh had the highest prevalence, 73% having arthrosis in one joint or other compared with 60% in the mean for all samples (P <.0005). Thirty percent had arthrosis in three or more joint groups compared with 22% in all samples (P < .0005). Wensleydale also had a rather high prevalence (P ≈.01) but it involved three or more joints in only 23%. The lowest prevalence in females (50%) was observed in the population of Tecumseh and Oberhörlen (P < .005 and .02). The three Indian populations had a low prevalence of the generalised form of osteoarthrosis (P < .05, < .01 and < .01 for 3+ joint groups) in the Haidas, Blackfeet and Pimas, in the Queen Charlotte Islands, Montana and Arizona.

Since the African, Czech and Swiss x-rays were read in 1967—72 they are compared with the 1967—72 readings of the other population samples in Figure 1. The data in Figure 1 is based on unweighted means of four age groups, those aged 65 plus being considered as one group. The prevalence was somewhat lower in this group because of the omission of the cervical spine; 50% of males and 57% of females aged 35 plus had osteoarthrosis in one joint or other compared

158

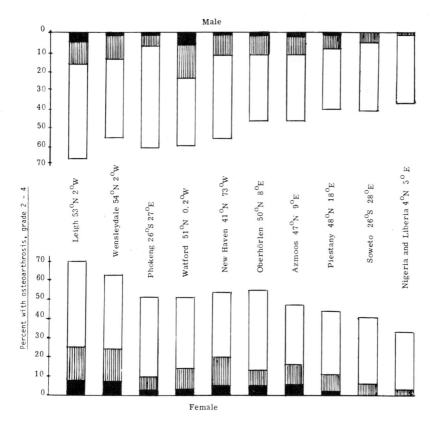

Figure 1   Osteoarthrosis in hands and feet in ten population samples aged 35+ (read 1967–72). Black = 5+; striped = 3–4; white = 1–2 joint groups.

with 60% in the first group. As in the first group the greatest prevalence was observed in Leigh (P < .005) in both sexes but the Wensleydale females and the Watford males also had significantly more than the mean for all populations (P < .05). The lowest prevalence was observed in Nigeria and Liberia where only 38% of men and 34% of women had osteoarthrosis but the population samples in Piéstany and Soweto also showed a significantly reduced prevalence and this also applied to the Azmoos women but not significantly to the men and not in either sex to the generalised form. Generalised O.A. had a particularly low prevalence in both sexes in Nigeria and Liberia (P < .005) and a particularly high prevalence in females in Leigh and Wensleydale (P < .005). As in the first group there was in these ten population samples no obvious relationship to latitude or longitude. Most striking was the lack of generalised osteoarthrosis in the negro populations in Africa.

159

Heberden's Nodes

Data on Heberden's nodes are available in ten of the population samples. The greatest frequency of Heberden's nodes was found in the population of Watford, 32% of whom were affected, but 30% of the Blackfeet Indians in Montana and 26% of a Swiss population in Azmoos had nodes (Table III). In these three populations the prevalence was high in both sexes though greater in females as it was in all the other Caucasian populations, except possibly Azmoos. All the negro populations had a very low prevalence of Heberden's nodes, varying between 3 and 5%. Two other populations had a low prevalence, the population of Oberhörlen in Germany and the Pima Indians in Arizona. In Oberhörlen the prevalence was low in both sexes but in the Pimas only the women had less than

TABLE III   Heberden's Nodes in Population Samples

Site and age		Males		Females			Male and female	
	Total	Grade of idiopathic Heberden's nodes in per cent		Total	Grade of idiopathic Heberden's nodes in per cent			
		2–4	3–4		2–4	3–4	2–4	3–4
Wensleydale 35+	309	13.5	4.3	356	27*	11.7	21NS	8
Leigh 35+	536	17.3	4.8	608	24.8†	7.1	21NS	6
Montana 35+	523	26.2‡		408	34.6¶		30.4¶	
Arizona 35+	416	20		395	11†		16*	
Watford 35+	123	27	15	136	37‡	14.2	32¶	15
Rhondda 35–64	520	5	0.4					
55–64	178	11	1	172	30	5	20	3
Glamorgan 55–64				86	21	3.5		
Oberhörlen 35+	101	11	4	164	13*	3	12†	4
Azmoos 35+	181	25	3.6	205	26NS	11	26†	7
Jamaica 35–64	263	2.7	0	270	7.7†	1.5	5.2¶	0.8
Nigeria & Liberia 35+	224	5	1.9	230	8	4.5	3.2¶	3
Phokeng 35+	89	4.9		234	2.2		3.6¶	
All populations Unweighted mean 35+	4483	17.3		3436	21.3		19.3	
35–64	3962	10.0		2826	13.5		12	
55–64	897			797	26.7		22	

* .05 >P>.01   † P < .01   ‡ P < .001   ¶ P < .0001

Percentages are unweighted means of four age groups except in Jamaica, the Rhondda and Glamorgan.

160

expected. Indeed a feature of the Pima Indians was the reversal of the normal sex distribution, only 11% of the women having nodes, compared with 20% in the men (P ≈ .001).

Nodal and Non-nodal Generalised Osteoarthrosis

When generalised osteoarthrosis is divided into nodal and non-nodal forms it becomes apparent that it is the nodal form which is less frequent in Jamaicans (Figures 2 and 3). In Nigeria and Liberia on the other hand both forms are rare

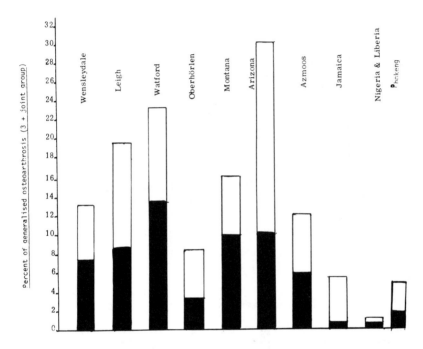

Figure 2   Nodal and non-nodal polyarthrosis aged 35+ except Jamaica (males).
Black = nodal; white = non-nodal.

(P < .0005). The greatest prevalence of nodal polyarthrosis was found in English women in Leigh, Wensleydale and Watford.

Non-nodal generalised O.A. was not significantly diminished in the Jamaican population but was greatly increased in the Pima males in Arizona, though not in the females.

In the Blackfeet Indians in Montana on the other hand the prevalence of non-nodal generalised O.A. was significantly less than expected in both sexes(P<.01), particularly in the older age groups.

161

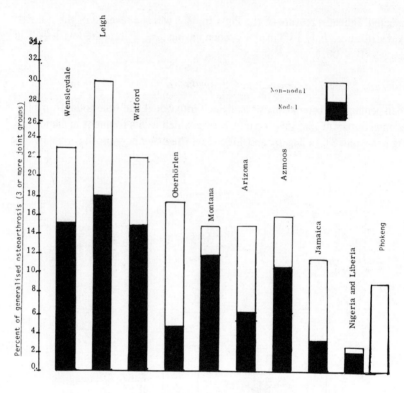

Figure 3   Nodal and non-nodal polyarthrosis aged 35+ except Jamaica (females).

Joint Pattern

Distal Interphalangeal (DIP) Joints

These were the most affected joints in eight of the 16 surveys (Table IV).
According to the 1963—5 readings they were affected in 34% of males and 39%
of females, a small but significant sex difference (P ≈ .001). Two surveys showed
exceptionally high frequencies in males, the Haida Indians in the Queen Charlotte
Islands (P < .05) and the Pima Indians in Arizona (P < .01). No excess however
was found in the Blackfeet Indians in Montana so that a racial influence is
improbable and it is more likely that occupational factors are responsible, fishing
in the Haidas and cotton growing in the Pimas. A feature of the x-ray findings in
the Haidas was that the osteophyte formation was not associated with any diminution of joint space suggesting that it is not true osteoarthrosis which is
responsible. An unusually low prevalence of osteoarthrosis in the DIP joints was
observed in the Wensleydale males, whose occupation is mainly sheep-farming
(P < .05).

162

TABLE IV   Radiological O.A. in DIP Joints of Fingers 1963–5 Readings

Site and age	Males Total	Males Grade of O.A. in per cent 2–4	Males Grade of O.A. in per cent 3–4	Females Total	Females Grade of O.A. in per cent 2–4	Females Grade of O.A. in per cent 3–4
Queen Charlotte Islands 35+ Unweighted mean	116	45†	0	93	36	7
Wensleydale 35+ Unweighted mean	293	25†	3	349	36	9
Leigh 35+ Unweighted mean	530	32	5	600	45†	9
Watford 35+ Unweighted mean	118	28	8	136	33	10
Oberhörlen (1963) 35+ Unweighted mean	112	26NS	4	147	31NS	7
Montana 35+ Unweighted mean	521	34	5	410	41	10
Tecumseh 35+ Unweighted mean	198	35	7	201	44NS	15
Arizona 35+ Unweighted mean	417	42‡	10	396	30‡	4
Jamaica 35–64 Unweighted mean	259	22	1	267	32	4
All Surveys Unweighted mean 35+	2564	34	6	2599	39	9
Unweighted mean 35–64	2079	23	1.9	2103	26	3.2

† $P < .05$ ‡ $P < .01$

In women osteoarthrosis of the DIP joints was more frequent than in men in all samples except the Haida and Pima Indians. The Pima women had significantly less than the women in other populations. The Leigh women on the other hand had significantly more than expected.

In the populations read in 1966–72 gradings tended to be lower (Table IVA). This was largely due to a change in interpretation of x-ray appearances in these joints, particularly in Jamaican x-rays. Apart from this the main feature of the x-rays read at this time was the low prevalence of osteoarthrosis of the DIP joints in the population of Nigeria and Liberia ($P < .0001$ in both sexes). This was confirmed in the Soweto females ($P < .01$), but was not significant in Phokeng

163

TABLE IVa   Radiological O.A. in DIP Joints of Fingers 1966–72 Readings

Site and age	Total	Grade of O.A. in per cent		Total	Grade of O.A. in per cent	
	(Males)	2–4	3–4	(Females)	2–4	3–4
Wensleydale 35+	293	23	2	349	31	8
Unweighted mean	293	23	2	349	31	8
Leigh 35+						
Unweighted mean	530	26	5	600	39†	9
Rhondda 35–64	514	12	2			
Unweighted mean 55–64				174	43	6
Watford 35+						
Unweighted mean	118	27	9	136	32	8
Oberhörlen 35+						
(1968 survey)						
Unweighted mean	101	17NS	2	164	30	4
Piéstany 35+						
Unweighted mean	505	23	4	574	32	4
Azmoos 35+						
Unweighted mean	189	18	3	225	29	8
New Haven 35+						
Unweighted mean	489	28	6	584	35	12
Jamaica 35–64						
Unweighted mean	259	12	1	267	25	2
Nigeria & Liberia						
Unweighted mean 35+	218	7¶	0.4	222	14¶	o.5
Phokeng 35+						
Unweighted mean	85	24	6	214	29NS	9
Soweto (Johannesburg)						
Unweighted mean 35+	80	15NS	4	168	23‡	5
All Surveys						
Unweighted mean 35+	3381	23	4.2	3677	34	7
Unweighted mean 35–64	2883	14	1.1	2912	20	2

† P ≈.03   ‡ P < .01   ¶ P < .0001

or in the other negro group in Jamaica. The highest prevalence was observed in females in Leigh (P ≈ .03), but none of the other populations showed a prevalence which was significantly greater than the mean for all populations.

Proximal Interphalangeal (PIP) Joints

Osteoarthrosis in these joints, as in the DIP joints was more frequent in women

164

TABLE V Radiological O.A. in PIP Joints of Fingers 1963–5 Readings

Site and age	Males			Females		
	Total	Grade of O.A. in per cent		Total	Grade of O.A. in per cent	
		2–4	3–4		2–4	3–4
Queen Charlotte Islands 35+						
Unweighted mean	119	21†	2	92	14	3
Wensleydale 35+						
Unweighted mean	293	8	1	349	16	4
Leigh 35+						
Unweighted mean	530	9	0.7	600	23‡	5
Watford 35+						
Unweighted mean	118	14	3	136	16	1
Oberhörlen 35+ (1963 survey)						
Unweighted mean	112	9	2	147	19	1
Montana 35+						
Unweighted mean	521	12	2	410	16	3
Tecumseh 35+						
Unweighted mean	198	18*	2	202	24†	9
Arizona 35+						
Unweighted mean	417	19‡	2	396	12†	1
Jamaica 35–64						
Unweighted mean	259	5	2	267	9	0.4
All Surveys						
Unweighted mean 35+	2567	13	2	2599	18	4
Unweighted mean 35–64	2082	7	0.7	2104	9	1

† P <.02   ‡ P < .005

in all populations with the exception of the Haida and Pima Indians (Table V). In the Haida Indians in the Queen Charlotte Islands the excess in males was limited to grade 2 which was present in 19% of males compared with a mean of 11% for males in all populations (P ≈ .02). Males in Arizona also had more osteoarthrosis in the PIP joints than females and more than the population mean (P < .005). A high prevalence in females was noted in Tecumseh and Leigh (P =.02 and < .01) and there was a low prevalence in the Arizona females (P ≈ .02).

In the second group (Table Va) there was no population in which males were more commonly affected and none of the males had an unusually high prevalence. A low prevalence was observed in Nigerian and Liberian males (P < .005), and in

TABLE Va Radiological O.A. in PIP Joints of Fingers 1966–72 Readings

Site and age	Males Total	Grade of O.A. in per cent 2–4	3–4	Females Total	Grade of O.A. in per cent 2–4	3–4
Wensleydale 35+ Unweighted mean	239	8	1	349	19	4
Leigh 35+ Unweighted mean	530	9	0.9	600	21	5
Rhondda 35–64	514	3	0.4			
Unweighted mean 55–64				174	19	3
Watford 35+ Unweighted mean	118	11	1	136	18	0.7
Oberhörlen 35+ (1968 survey Unweighted mean	101	10	2	164	17	1
Piéstany 35+ Unweighted mean	505	9	0.7	574	14	3
Azmoos 35+ Unweighted mean	189	10	1	225	19	5
New Haven 35+ Unweighted mean	490	7	0.7	584	18	4
Jamaica 35+ Unweighted mean	259	4	1	267	7	0
Nigeria & Liberia Unweighted mean 35+	218	3	0.7	222	8	0.5
Phokeng 35+ Unweighted mean	86	7	0.7	214	10†	0.3
Soweto 35+ Unweighted mean	80	7	1	168	9	2
All Surveys Unweighted mean 35+	3383	8	1	3677	17	3
Unweighted mean 35–64	2484	4	0.4	2949	8	0.8

† P < .005

all the African female populations. The Jamaicans, though of African stock, did not show the same low prevalence. None of the female populations in the second group had an exceptionally high prevalence.

Metacarpophalangeal (MCP) Joints

The MCP joints did not show the same female predominance (Table VI). Indeed

TABLE VI   Radiological O.A. in MCP Joints 1963–5 Readings

Site and age		Males			Females		
		Total	Grade of O.A. in per cent		Total	Grade of O.A. in per cent	
			2–4	3–4		2–4	3–4
Queen Charlotte Islands 35+ Unweighted mean		119	15	5	93	11	0
Wensleydale 35+ Unweighted mean		293	16*	2	349	22‡	5
Leigh 35+ Unweighted mean		530	18	5	600	17	2
Watford 35+ Unweighted mean		118	22	3	135	20	2
Oberhörlen 35+ (1963 survey) Unweighted mean		112	12	3	147	16	2
Montana 35+ Unweighted mean		521	18	2	410	10	0.6
Tecumseh 35+ Unweighted mean		198	17	7	202	15	5
Arizona 35+ Unweighted mean		417	42¶	17¶	396	11	1
Jamaica 35–64 Unweighted mean		259	11	0.9	267	9	0
All Surveys Unweighted mean 35+		2567	24	6	2599	16	3
Unweighted mean 35–64		2082	17	2		8	0.5

* P ≈ .05   ‡ P < .005   ¶ P < .0001

in the first group the males had significantly more (P < .0001). As in the inter-phalangeal joints the Arizona males had an exceptionally high prevalence (42%) (P < .0001) and it applied to all grades of severity. In contradistinction to the interphalangeal joints the females in Arizona showed no excess, suggesting that an occupational influence is responsible for the exceptional MCP involvement in males. A low prevalence (12%) was observed in the Oberhörlen males (P≈.04) but not in the females. The Wensleydale males also had little involvement (16% – P ≈ .05), but the females had more than expected (P < .005).

In the second group of readings (Table VIa) only the Watford sample showed an excessive prevalence in both sexes (P < .01 in men and ≈ .01 in women) but the rather high prevalence in females in Wensleydale becomes significant in this

TABLE VIa   Radiological O.A. in MCP Joints 1966–72 Readings

Site and age	Males Total	Grade of O.A. in per cent 2–4	Grade of O.A. in per cent 3–4	Females Total	Grade of O.A. in per cent 2–4	Grade of O.A. in per cent 3–4
Wensleydale 35+ Unweighted mean	293	16	1	349	22¶	3
Leigh 35+ Unweighted mean	530	17	4	600	15	2
Rhondda 35–64 Unweighted mean 55–64	514	6†	2	174	14	2
Watford 35+ Unweighted mean	118	23‡	5	135	22†	2
Oberhörlen 35+ (1968 survey) Unweighted mean	101	13	2	164	14	0.6
Piéstany 35+ Unweighted mean	505	10	2	574	15	1
Azmoos 35+ Unweighted mean	189	12	3	225	13	2
New Haven 35+ Unweighted mean	490	11	1	584	9‡	0.7
Jamaica 35–64 Unweighted mean	259	9	0.6	267	7	0
Nigeria & Liberia 35+ Unweighted mean	218	5‡	2	222	2¶	0
Phokeng 35+ Unweighted mean	86	19NS	4	214	9*	0.9
Soweto 35+ Unweighted mean	80	8NS	2	168	11	4
All Surveys Unweighted mean 35+	3383	13	3	3676	14	1
Unweighted mean 35–64	2885	8	0.9	2949	7	0.5

* P ≈ .04   † P ≈ .01   ‡ P < .01   ¶ P < .0005

reading (P < .0005). The lowest prevalence was found in Nigeria and Liberia where only 5% of men and 2% of women had osteoarthrosis in this joint (P < .001). The Rhondda males also had a rather low prevalence (P ≈ .01) and also the Phokeng (P ≈ .04) and New Haven females (P < .005).

The Carpo-metacarpal (CMC) Joints

Osteoarthrosis was practically limited to the first joint. This is an important joint, since it is predominantly involved in the nodal form of generalised OA.

No significant differences were observed between the male samples apart from Oberhörlen and Montana which had a low prevalence (P ≈ .05 and < .01), but in females a high prevalence was observed in Leigh (P < .005) (Table VII). The females in Wensleydale, Watford and Tecumseh also showed a rather high prevalence. Because of the small numbers examined it was not significant. Thus all the Caucasian females apart from those in Oberhörlen had a relatively high prevalence of arthrosis in the first CMC joints. By contrast all the Indian females

TABLE VII   Radiological O.A. in CMC Joints 1963–5 Readings

Site and age		Males			Females		
		Total	Grade of O.A. in per cent		Total	Grade of O.A. in per cent	
			2–4	3–4		2–4	3–4
Queen Charlotte Islands 35+ Unweighted mean		119	8	2	93	7	0
Wensleydale 35+ Unweighted mean		293	13	2	349	17NS	5
Leigh 35+ Unweighted mean		529	15	5	600	20¶	5
Watford 35+ Unweighted mean		118	16NS	8	135	18NS	5
Oberhörlen 35+ (1963 survey) Unweighted mean		112	5*	1	147	11	5
Montana 35+ Unweighted mean		520	7‡	0.1	410	6	1
Tecumseh 35+ Unweighted mean		198	15	4	202	18NS	6
Arizona 35+ Unweighted mean		417	13	3	396	9†	1
Jamaica 35–64 Unweighted mean		259	6	0	267	3†	0
All surveys Unweighted mean 35+		2565	12	3	2599	14	4
Unweighted mean 35–64		2080	6	0.7	2104	8	1

* P ≈ .05   † P ≈ .02   ‡ P < .01   ¶ P < .005

TABLE VIIa   Radiological O.A. in CMC Joints 1967–72 Readings

Site and age	Males Total	Males Grade of O.A. in per cent 2–4	Males Grade of O.A. in per cent 3–4	Females Total	Females Grade of O.A. in per cent 2–4	Females Grade of O.A. in per cent 3–4
Wensleydale 35+ Unweighted mean	293	13†	1	349	17‡	5
Leigh 35+ Unweighted mean	529	12†	4	600	17‡	5
Rhondda 35–64	514	4	0.6			
Unweighted mean 55–64				174	22	4
Watford 35+ Unweighted mean	118	16	8	135	18†	5
Oberhörlen (1968) 35+ Unweighted mean	101	5	1	164	9	3
Piéstany 35+ Unweighted mean	505	5	0.7	574	8†	2
Azmoos 35+ Unweighted mean	189	6	1	225	12	4
New Haven 35+ Unweighted mean	490	8	0.8	584	13	3
Jamaica 35–64 Unweighted mean	259	3†	0.9	267	2†	0
Nigeria & Liberia 35+ Unweighted mean	218	3‡	0	222	1¶	0
Phokeng 35+ Unweighted mean	86	8	1	213	3¶	0.3
Soweto 35+ Unweighted mean	80	6	1	167	2¶	0.4
All Surveys Unweighted mean 35+	3382	8	2	3674	11	3
Unweighted mean 35–64		4	0.4	2948	6	1

† P ≈ .02   ‡ P < .01   ¶ P < .0005

had a low prevalence varying from 6% in Montana (P < .0005) to 9% in Arizona (P ≈ .04). A low prevalence was also noted in the Jamaican females (P ≈ .02).

In the second group (Table VIIa) the population of Watford had the greatest prevalence of osteoarthrosis in the CMC joints, 16% in males (P < .005) and 18% in females (P ≈ .02), but the other two English populations also had a significant excess, particularly the females (P < .01). This however did not apply to the

Welsh population in the Rhondda which had slightly below the average. Nor did it apply to the German, Swiss or Czechoslovak population. Indeed the Czechoslovak sample had significantly less than the mean (P ≈ .04 in the women). The lowest frequencies however were found in the negro women, all of whom had significantly less than the mean. The negro males also had less than expected in Nigeria and Jamaica, though the difference was less striking.

Wrists

There were no geographical differences in the prevalence of osteoarthrosis of the wrists in males in the first group, but females in the Queen Charlotte Islands had a rather high prevalence (P ≈ .03) (Table VIII). In the second group (Table VIIIa)

TABLE VIII   Radiological O.A. in Wrist 1963–5 Readings

Site and age	Males			Females		
	Total	Grade of O.A. in per cent		Total	Grade of O.A. in per cent	
		2–4	3–4		2–4	3–4
Queen Charlotte Islands 35+ Unweighted mean	118	12	4	93	10	5
Wensleydale 35+ Unweighted mean	290	8	2	348	7	2
Leigh 35+ Unweighted mean	526	10	1	595	5	0.3
Watford 35+ Unweighted mean	117	13	4	135	6	0
Oberhörlen 35+ (1963 survey) Unweighted mean	111	6	2	147	3	0
Montana 35+ Unweighted mean	514	11	3	409	3	0.6
Tecumseh 35+ Unweighted mean	197	7	2	201	6	1
Arizona 35+ Unweighted mean	415	11	2	396	4	0.7
Jamaica 35+ Unweighted mean	259	5	0.8	267	3	0.8
All Surveys Unweighted mean 35+	2547	10	2	2591	5	0.8
Unweighted mean 35–64	2069	6	1	2099	3	0.5

TABLE VIIIa   Radiological O.A. in Wrist 1967–72 Readings

Site and age	Total	Grade of O.A. in per cent		Total	Grade of O.A. in per cent	
		2–4	3–4		2–4	3–4
Wensleydale 35+ Unweighted mean	390	11	2	346	7†	0.8
Leigh 35+ Unweighted mean	526	10	3	595	4	0.6
Rhondda 35+ Unweighted mean	483	6	1	174	6	3
Watford 35+ Unweighted mean	117	10	3	135	6	0
Oberhörlen 35+ (1968 survey) Unweighted mean	101	7	2	164	5	0
Piéstany 35+ Unweighted mean	499	7	0.9	571	3	0.4
Azmoos 35+ Unweighted mean	189	1‡	0	220	1†	0
New Haven 35+ Unweighted mean	483	8	1	581	3	0.2
Jamaica 35–64 Unweighted mean	259	4	1	267	3	0.7
Nigeria & Liberia 35+ Unweighted mean	218	5	0	222	7†	0.5
Phokeng (Tswanas) 35+ Unweighted mean	81	6	0	210	4	0.6
Soweto 35+ Unweighted mean	80	8	4	162	3	0.5
All Surveys Unweighted mean 35+	3356	8	2	3647	4	0.6
Unweighted mean 35–64	2865	5	0.9	2936	2	0.4

† P ≈ .03   ‡ P < .005

the population of Azmoos had an exceptionally low prevalence in both sexes (P < .005 in males and P ≈ .03 in females). A rather high prevalence was noted in the Wensleydale (P ≈ .02) and Nigerian and Liberian females (P ≈ .02).

Hips

Osteoarthrosis of the hips has been assessed from the age of 55 since in some

172

surveys the hips were not x-rayed in the younger age groups (Table IX). The prevalence in the combined populations aged 55+ was 14% in males and 13% in females, in the first group 17% and 10% in the second (Table IXa), a significant difference in the latter ($P \approx .0001$). The sex relationship varied greatly in different

TABLE IX   Radiological O.A. hips 1963–5 Readings

Site and age		Males			Females		
		Total	Grade of O.A. in per cent		Total	Grade of O.A. in per cent	
			2–4	3–4		2–4	3–4
Queen Charlotte Islands Unweighted mean	55+	36	7	3			
Wensleydale Unweighted mean	55+	102	22*	12	149	18	10
Leigh Unweighted mean	55+	236	22‡	8	265	14	5
Watford 55+ Unweighted mean		39	10	6	38	9	2
Montana Unweighted mean	55+	144	8	3	98	11	4
Arizona Unweighted mean	55+	162	12	2	105	5	0.8
Jamaica Unweighted mean	55–64	86	2‡	0	79	4	0
All Surveys Unweighted mean	55+	805	14	6	734	13	5

* $P \approx .04$ ‡ $P < .01$

populations. A relatively high prevalence was noted in the males in Wensleydale ($P \approx .04$) and Leigh ($P < .01$) and a low prevalence in both sexes in Jamaica ($P < .01$), Liberia and Nigeria ($P < .005$) and Phokeng ($P < .01$). The differences were more noticeable in the males.

TABLE IXa   Radiological O.A. Hips 1967—72 Readings

Site and age		Males			Females		
		Total	Grade of O.A. in per cent		Total	Grade of O.A. in per cent	
			2—4	3—4		2—4	3—4
Wensleydale 55+ Unweighted mean		102	22	9	149	16	11
Leigh 55+ Unweighted mean		236	25‡	7	265	15	5
Watford 55+ Unweighted mean		39	12	4	38	7	0
Oberhörlen 55+ (1968 survey) Unweighted mean		50	16	6	69	10	5
Piestany 55+		180	17	3	196	10	3
Azmoos 55+ Unweighted mean		93	17	7	130	7	4
Jamaica 55—64 Unweighted mean		87	1‡	0	91	4	4
Nigeria & Liberia 55+ Unweighted mean		66	3‡	2	60	2NS	0.9
Phokeng 55+ Unweighted mean		61	3‡	1	138	3‡	0
All Surveys Unweighted mean 55+		914	17	6	1136	10	4
Unweighted mean 55—64		576	14	4	664	8	2

‡ P < .01

Knees

X-rays of the knees were performed in only five of the population samples. The prevalence in these five samples was 19% in males and 30% in females, a very significant difference which was present in all five surveys (P < .0001) (Table X). A low prevalence was noted in the Wensleydale males, only 14% of whom had any evidence of osteoarthrosis in the knees (P ≈ .03), but the Wensleydale

174

TABLE X   Radiological O.A. Knees 1967–72 Readings

Site and age	Males Total	Males Grade of O.A. in per cent 2–4	Males Grade of O.A. in per cent 3–4	Females Total	Females Grade of O.A. in per cent 2–4	Females Grade of O.A. in per cent 3–4
Leigh 35+						
Unweighted mean	512	21	4	580	31	10
Wensleydale 35+						
Unweighted mean	286	14†	2	345	28	10
Watford 35+						
Unweighted mean	118	19	5	129	24NS	7
Jamaica 35–64						
Unweighted mean	256	19*	3	255	28†	7
Piestany 35+						
Unweighted mean	371	17	3	433	23†	5
All Surveys						
Unweighted mean 35+	1543	19	4	1742	30	8
Unweighted mean 35–64	1289	14	2	1381	21	5

NS P > .05   * P ≈ .04   † P = .02 − .03

females did not have significantly less than the mean for all populations. The Jamaicans had rather higher frequencies than expected in both sexes (P ≈ .03).

First Metatarsophalangeal (MTP) Joints

Involvement of these joints came second in frequency to the DIP joints of the fingers (Table XI). They were more commonly affected in females (P < .0001). A very high prevalence of osteoarthrosis in the first MTP joints was a feature of the two urban populations in the United Kingdom. In Leigh 45% of males aged 35 and over were affected (P < .0005), in Watford 50% (P < .0005) compared with 28% in the total group. A low prevalence was noted in the Indian populations, notably in the Queen Charlotte Islands, where only 9% of males and 15% of females had osteoarthrosis in these joints (P < .0005 and .001). An exception is the Arizona males who had roughly the expected amount. A low prevalence was observed in the Jamaican males.

The second group of readings (Table XIa) confirms the high prevalence in the two urban populations in the United Kingdom. As in the first group only females in Wensleydale had a high prevalence. The low prevalence in Jamaicans is also

175

TABLE XI   Osteoarthrosis 1st MTP Joints 1963–5 Readings

	Males			Females		
Site and age	Total	Grade of O.A. in per cent		Total	Grade of O.A. in per cent	
		2–4	3–4		2–4	3–4
Queen Charlotte Islands 35+						
Unweighted mean	119	9¶	1	93	15‡	0
Wensleydale 35+						
Unweighted mean	289	27	6	350	43†	9
Leigh 35+						
Unweighted mean	527	45¶	11	597	54¶	12
Watford 35+						
Unweighted mean	118	50¶	17	133	42NS	12
Oberhörlen 35+ (1963 survey)						
Unweighted mean	111	24	1	147	14	1
Montana 35+						
Unweighted mean	519	16¶	2	408	16¶	1
Arizona 35+						
Unweighted mean	418	29	4	396	24¶	1
Jamaica 35–64						
Unweighted mean	258	16‡	0.8	268	28NS	2
All surveys 35+						
Unweighted mean 35+	2359	28¶	6	2392	36¶	7
Unweighted mean 35–64	1923	25	4	1952	33	5

‡ P < .001   ¶ P < .0005

confirmed and all the negro populations show a low prevalence in both sexes. The lowest prevalence however is observed in the Piéstany sample, only 9% of whom are affected (P < .0001). The population of Azmoos also had less than the expected amount (P < .0005).

The pattern of osteoarthrosis in different populations is compared in Figures 4–6. The most striking feature is the frequent involvement of the first MTP joints in the English populations. The American Indian populations on the other hand show predominant involvement of the distal interphalageal joints of the

TABLE XIa   Radiological Osteoarthrosis 1st MTP Joints 1967–72 Readings

Site and age		Males			Females		
		Total	Grade of O.A. in per cent		Total	Grade of O.A. in per cent	
			2–4	3–4		2–4	3–4
Queen Charlotte Islands							
Wensleydale Unweighted mean	35+	289	31NS	7	350	41‡	8
Leigh Unweighted mean	35+	527†	47¶	10	597	49¶	12
Rhondda Unweighted mean	55–64	514	25	4	174	44	13
Watford Unweighted mean	35+	118	43‡	13	133	36NS	12
Oberhörlen (1968 survey) Unweighted mean	35+	101	27	0	164	19	1
Piestany Unweighted mean	35+	504	9¶	1	573	9¶	1
Azmoos Unweighted mean	35+	189	16¶	2	225	19¶	0.9
New Haven Unweighted mean	35+	488	29NS	9	585	30	13
Jamaica Unweighted mean	35–64	258	17†	0.8‡	264	27	0.8†
Nigeria & Liberia Unweighted mean	35+	217	15†	0.5	220	16‡	0
Phokeng Unweighted mean	35+	87	15*	2	212	18‡	2
Soweto Unweighted mean	35+	81	15*	5	170	17†	3
All surveys (1967–72)	35+	3373	26	5	3667	29	5
	35–64	2877	23	4	2939	26	4

*P ≈ .05   † P < .01   ‡ P < .005   ¶ P < .0001

177

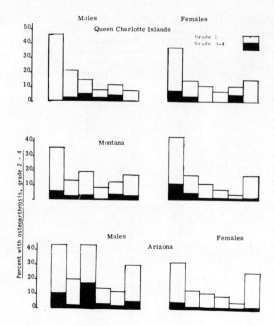

Figure 4 Pattern of osteoarthrosis in American Indians (aged 35+)

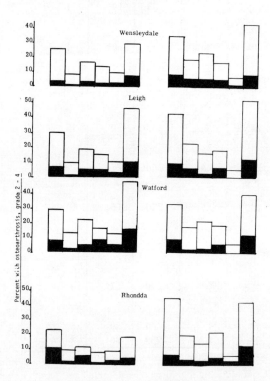

Figure 5 Pattern of osteoarthrosis in UK populations (aged 35+)

178

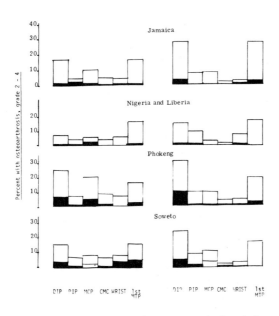

Figure 6   Pattern of osteoarthrosis in Negroes (aged 35+, except Jamaica).

fingers but the males in Arizona also have frequent involvement of the MCP joints. The negroes tend to have less frequent involvement of all joints.

Discussion

The factors influencing the prevalence of osteoarthrosis in populations are clearly very complex depending on occupation, heredity and possibly diet and resultant body build. Climate is often blamed for rheumatic troubles but there is no evidence from the present study that it influences the prevalence of osteo-arthrosis. It is true that the lowest prevalence was found in the samples in Nigeria and Liberia at 40°N and the highest in Leigh at 53°N, but Jamaica at 18°N had a greater prevalence than the Haida Indians in the Queen Charlotte Islands at 54°N and there is in general no relationship to latitude.

Where there is disparity between the sexes and where males show a relatively high prevalence, as for example in Arizona, an occupational influence must be presumed. In this population 1% of males had osteoarthrosis in five or more joint groups, more than twice the population mean whereas females had only half the expected amount ($P < .0001$). Heberden's nodes were also more common in Pima men (Bennett & Burch, 1968). The men are concerned mainly with farming, cotton being an important product. It is perhaps of interest that an occupational influence predisposing to the development of Heberden's nodes has

179

so far been found by us only in cotton spinners and weavers (Lawrence, 1961).

The high prevalence of osteoarthrosis in the DIP joints in the Leigh women may well depend partly on their occupation, since most women in Leigh work in the textile mills, an occupation which is known to affect the finger joints, particularly the DIP joints. This is consistent with the high prevalence of nodal generalised OA already noted in this group and with the high frequency of nodal generalised OA in textile workers (Lawrence, 1961). A high prevalence was also present in the Tecumseh women, particularly of the more severe grades. Many of the women worked in a large factory manufacturing compression engines for refrigerators. In Watford also it was chiefly the males who had an excessive prevalence of generalised osteoarthrosis but there was no obvious occupational influence. Those with generalised arthrosis and Heberden's nodes were mainly clerks or machine operators. There is no evidence that these occupations influence the pattern of osteoarthrosis.

It is difficult to escape the conclusion that racial differences play a large part in determining predisposition to generalised osteoarthrosis. The American Indians appear to have a distinct advantage from this point of view. In all three Indian samples the women had significantly less osteoarthrosis in three or more joint groups than expected. Apart from those in Montana this did not apply to the male Indians. The Haida Indians are fishermen. A distinct tendency to develop generalised osteoarthrosis has been noted in another group of fishermen in North Germany (Behrend et al, 1977). In this population also it was mainly the distal interphalangeal joints of the fingers which were involved, but involvement of these joints is a feature of all Amerindian populations. In the Pima males, the MCP joints were also commonly affected but this was probably occupational since the females did not show this feature.

The low prevalence of generalised osteoarthrosis and particularly of osteoarthrosis of the DIP and CMC joints, in the negro populations in Africa is consistent with Stechner's (1940) finding of infrequent Heberden's nodes in American negroes seen in hospital practice and the findings of Muller (1970), Muller et al, (1972) and Solomon and Beighton (1975) in African negroes. Beighton found Heberden's nodes to be frequent (37%) in a population of part English ancestry in Tristan da Cunha. Our Jamaican population had more generalised osteoarthrosis than the other negro samples but lacked Heberden's nodes. This is consistent with the high prevalence of sero-negative polyarthritis in this population (Lawrence et al, 1966). Similarly the low prevalence of generalised osteoarthrosis in the negro populations in Nigeria and Liberia and also in Czechoslovakia is consistent with their low prevalence of sero-negative polyarthritis (Muller 1970; Sebo & Sitaj, 1968).

Caucasians show considerable variation in the frequency of Heberden's nodes, even in females, but this is not surprising in view of their very mixed origin. The nodal form of generalised osteoarthrosis is more frequent in the English females than any others. It is less common in the Welsh populations in the Rhondda and

Glamorgan. The Rhondda and Glamorgan populations are mainly Celtic stock and may originally have come from central Europe in migrations occurring in the second millenium BC (McEveda, 1967). They have mixed little with descendants of later Anglo-Saxon and Viking migrations of Teutonic stock.

Kellgren in his original description of the nodal form of generalised osteoarthrosis (Kellgren & Moore, 1952) noted the frequent involvement of the first CMC joint in this condition. It is therefore of interest that this joint was less affected in the American Indian and Negro females and more affected in the English females.

Though the first MTP joint is affected more in persons with Heberden's nodes and reflects the racial distribution of nodal osteoarthrosis in females, the relatively high frequency of osteoarthrosis in this joint in the English populations is quite out of proportion and suggests that other factors are operative. One possibility is that faulty footwear may be responsible. With this in view we are at present looking at the frequency of hallux valgus in these population samples. The Welsh males in the Rhondda were relatively free of osteoarthrosis in this joint. They are mainly miners and wear boots specifically designed to protect the toes.

Comparison of our findings with those of Roberts and Burch (1966) derived from the US National Health Survey indicate similar prevalences to those we have found; unweighted means for rural females aged 35+ in 1+ joints being 56% for whites and 47% for negroes. Figures for generalised osteoarthrosis are not given but grade 3–4 osteoarthrosis in the hands or feet was present in 20% of whites and 9% of negroes. In males the difference was less striking, 14% in whites and 11% in negroes.

Comparison with the readings of Bennett and Burch (1968) on the Blackfeet and Pima Indians shows that they graded arthrosis at a higher level than we have done, our grade 2–4 being intermediate between their grade 2–4 and 3–4. Such interobserver differences are to be expected and stress the importance of having all samples read by the same observer, when comparison between populations is to be made. Their conclusion that there is a greater prevalence of osteoarthrosis in Arizona males than in females is in agreement with ours.

The difference between Pima and Blackfeet males was in the non-nodal type. A high fluoride content was reported in some wells on the Pima reservation and several investigators have reported that fluoride aggravates the manifestations of osteoarthrosis. In mice, Zipkin, Sokoloff and Frazier (1967) found no influence from fluoride over a period of 15 months at a level of 50 parts per million in the drinking water. It is unlikely that fluoride could be responsible for the greater prevalence of osteoarthrosis in Pima males since the females showed no excess.

Sherman (1943) noticed that Indians were relatively insensitive to pain and this might be thought to predispose to osteoarthrosis after the manner of a Charcot joint but only one tribe showed an excessive prevalence of osteoarthrosis and this only in one sex.

Summary

Skeletal x-rays from 16 random or area population samples, aged 35 and over, comprising Caucasians, Negroes and American Indians, have been graded for osteoarthrosis in two batches by a single observer. The first batch comprised 6165 individuals and the second 7050, 941 persons being present in both batches.

The highest prevalence of osteoarthrosis in both batches was found in the population of Leigh in the north of England where 67% of males and 73% of females had arthrosis in one or more joints. In general the English populations had more than any other, and the lowest prevalence was observed in Nigeria and Liberia. In Soweto in South Africa and in Piestany in Czechoslovakia the prevalence was also low. There was no consistent relationship to latitude or longitude. Generalised osteoarthrosis of the nodal type was rare in the negroes, but very common in the English populations particularly the women.

The pattern of joint involvement differed considerably in different populations. In the English populations the first metatarsophalangeal joints were most frequently affected, particularly in urban populations. A low prevalence in these joints was noted in the American Indian populations and also in Negroes. All the Caucasian populations apart from that in the Rhondda had a high prevalence of osteoarthrosis in the first carpometacarpal joints in females whereas the Indian and Negroe females had a low prevalence in this joint.

Osteoarthrosis of the hips was particularly common in males in the north of England where 22 to 25% of males aged 55 and over were affected. These were mainly coalminers and shepherds. It was rare in all Negro populations; only 1 to 3% of Negro men and 2 to 4% of women were affected. Osteoarthrosis of the knees affected mainly women and was more frequent in Jamaicans.

It is concluded that wide geographical differences exist affecting both the prevalence of osteoarthrosis and the pattern of joint involvement. Race influences particularly the prevalence of generalised arthrosis and more especially the form associated with Heberden's nodes.

References

Atlas of Standard Radiographs of Arthritis (1963). In *The Epidemiology of Chronic Rheumatism, Vol.II,* Blackwell, Oxford. Page 2

Beighton, PH, Solomon, L and Valkenburg, H (1975) *Annals of the Rheumatic Diseases, 34,* 136

Bennett, PH and Burch, TAB (1968). In *Population Studies of the Rheumatic Diseases.* Exerpta Medica Foundation, Amsterdam. Page 407

Bennett, PH and Wood, PHN (1968). In *Population Studies of the Rheumatic Diseases.* Exerpta Medica Foundation, Amsterdam. Page 465

Blumberg, BS, Bloch, KJ, Black, RL and Dotter, C (1961) *Arthritis and Rheumatism, 4,* 325

Kellgren, JH, Jeffrey, MR and Ball, J (1963). In *The Epidemiology of Chronic Rheumatism, Vol.II.* Blackwell, Oxford

Kellgren, JH and Moore, R (1952) *British Medical Journal, 1,* 181

Lawrence, JS (1961) *British Journal of Industrial Medicine, 18,* 270

Lawrence, JS (1977) *Rheumatism in Populations, chapter V, figs. 5.1 to 5.9.*
Wm Heinemann Medical Publications, London. Page 100
Lawrence, JS, de Graaf, R and Laine, VAJ (1963). In *The Epidemiology of Chronic
Rheumatism.* (Ed) JH Kellgren, M Jeffrey and J Ball. Blackwell, Oxford. Page 108
McEvedy, C (1967). *The Penguin Atlas of Ancient History.* Penguin Books, Harmondsworth,
England. Page 28
Muller, AS (1970) *Population Studies on the Prevalence of Rheumatic Diseases in Liberia
and Nigeria.* JH Pasmans, The Hague. Page 4
Muller, AS, Valkenburg, HA and Greenwood, BM (1972) *East African Medical Journal,
49,* 75
Roberts, J and Burch, TA (1966) *O.A. Prevalence in Adults.* US Department of Health,
Education and Welfare, National Centre for Health Statistics. Series 11 no.15, Page 18
Sebo, M and Sitaj, S (1968) *Bratislavski Lekarske Listy, 49,* 510
Sherman, ED (1943) *Canadian Medical Association Journal, 48,* 437
Sitaj, S and Sebo, M (1968). In *Population Studies of the Rheumatic Diseases.*
(Ed) PH Bennett and PHN Wood, Exerpta Medica Foundation, Amsterdam. Page 64
Solomon, L, Beighton, P and Lawrence, JS (1975) *South African Medical Journal, 49,* 1737
Solomon, L, Robin, G and Valkenburg, HA (1975) *Annals of the Rheumatic Diseases,
34,* 128
Stecher, R (1940) *New England Journal of Medicine, 222,* 300
Zinn, WM (1970) *Annals of Physical Medicine, 10,* 209
Zipkin, I, Sokoloff, L and Frazier, PD (1967) *Israel Journal of Medical Sciences, 3,* 719

17

GENETIC FACTORS IN OSTEOARTHROSIS

P Harper and G Nuki

Introduction

The study of the genetic contribution to the pathogenesis of human osteoarthrosis has been approached in a variety of ways and has yielded results which have not always been easy to interpret. This article attempts to clarify some of the discrepancies, to illustrate the value and limitations of the different types of study, and to indicate where opportunities may lie for advancing our knowledge.

One major line of approach has been to take patients with osteoarthrosis in a specific population and to analyse the frequency and form of the disease in relatives. Such an approach is essentially an extension of the more general epidemiological approach that has provided valuable information on both environmental and genetic factors. Both the approach and the results are quantitative, and contribute more to an assessment of the *importance* of genetic factors than to their *nature*. Attempts to identify these individual genetic factors from population studies have relied on the search for associations with recognised hereditary characters such as blood group and other genetic markers (Stoia et al, 1967; Lawrence, 1977).

The alternative approach has been to utilise models of osteoarthrosis in the hope that they will prove simpler to understand than the heterogeneous mass of degenerative joint disease in the population as a whole where multiple aetiological factors are operative. Such models may be provided by arthritis occurring in experimental animals, or by those naturally occurring human diseases, the rare genetic disorders, in which arthritis is a major manifestation of the clinical picture. This chapter deliberately emphasises the value of this last approach, not because the others have been fruitless, but because it has been under-valued and because it offers the most promising way of identifying the molecular bases for the pathogenesis of osteoarthrosis as well as the mechanisms responsible for normal development and continued function of joints.

Assessment of the Genetic Component of Human Osteoarthrosis

Although the early studies of Stecher (1941, 1955) recognised the familial occurrence of Heberden's nodes, it was not until the study of Kellgren and Moore (1952) that it became clear that in some cases of Heberden's nodes there was an associated generalised joint disease, termed by them primary generalised osteoarthritis. Attempts to distinguish this from other forms of osteoarthrosis led to systematic family studies being carried out and extensive data are now available from the epidemiological studies of Kellgren, Lawrence and colleagues performed in Northern England (Kellgren et al, 1963; Lawrence, 1977). The careful use of control data and the accurate clinical and radiological grading of abnormalities greatly enhances the value of this information, as does the completeness of their samples, extending and confirming earlier work which had suggested an increase in degenerative joint disease in first degree relatives (Hermann, 1936).

The results of these studies clearly show that Heberden's nodes apart, generalised osteoarthrosis does not follow simple Mendelian inheritance, whether or not it is associated with Heberden's nodes. Among first degree relatives, both sexes showed double the expected prevalence of arthritis, this being more severe though not more common in relatives of those probands with Heberden's nodes. No evidence was found of a common genetic predisposition to osteoarthrosis and rheumatoid arthritis, and no increase of osteoarthrosis in spouses occurred. These results fit well with those to be expected on the basis of polygenic inheritance, but a piece of information that is at present lacking for generalised osteoarthrosis is whether the risk in relatives is dependent on the sex of the proband. For polygenic disorders showing a marked variation in frequency between the sexes, a higher risk is to be expected among relatives of a proband of the more rarely affected sex, and a difference might be expected in this respect between the relatives of nodal and non-nodal cases if, as is suggested, they represent genetically different entities.

The apportionment of relative importance to genetic and environmental factors is generally a fruitless task unless these factors can be specifically identified, and although estimates of 'heritability' can be calculated (Falconer, 1965; Carter, 1969), they are generally approximate and may give a false sense of exactness to a situation which is often genuinely complicated by genetic heterogeneity and by familial influences which are not necessarily genetic. Twin studies can give an approximate indication of the importance of genetic factors, and such evidence as exists (King, 1968; Lawrence, 1977) shows a marked excess of concordance in monozygotic as opposed to dizygotic twin pairs which supports the prominent role of genetic factors.

While the types of study discussed above are valuable in demonstrating the role of inheritance in a common and variable disorder such as osteoarthrosis they are unable to identify the individual genes that are contributing to this role, and for this a different approach is needed. In part, this can be achieved by the study of osteoarthrosis in the general population in relation to known genetic variables, but in large measure a more indirect approach is needed. The approach is from the study of those models

185

provided by specific forms of arthritis in experimental animals and in the rarer
human Mendelian disorders where arthritis forms an integral part.

The Identification of Individual Genes in Generalised Osteoarthrosis

As yet we are unable to identify any one of the multiple genetic factors that it is
clear from family studies are involved in human osteoarthrosis. The distribution of
ABO and Rh blood groups has been studied in both Northern England and the
Rhondda, South Wales and no difference found from the general population frequencies (Lawrence, 1977). Other genetic markers have not been studied and in
particular there is little data as yet on HLA types in relation to osteoarthrosis.
Although there is no reason to implicate the HLA region in osteoarthrosis, the strik
associations found between particular HLA phenotypes and such disorders as anky-
losing spondylitis show how valuable such a discovery would be. There seems little
doubt that the HLA region is directly involved in the pathogenesis of this disease,
and whereas before this discovery the family data had a nondescript appearance of
polygenic inheritance somewhat similar to that seen in osteoarthrosis, the situation
has now been transformed with the HLA phenotype forming a valuable aid in pre-
diction of individuals at risk. Unfortunately, the distribution of HLA A and B locus
antigens in patients with osteoarthrosis of the small joints of the hands does not
differ from that in the general population (Ercilla et al, 1977).

Heberden's Nodes

There is general agreement that this common abnormality shows a strong familial
tendency, is more frequent in women and is associated with more general osteoarthrosis in some individuals (Kellgren and Moore, 1952). The precise model of
inheritance and the nature of the relationship with osteoarthrosis are less clearly
defined. Stecher (1941) was the first to study the genetic aspects, and showed that
among the relatives of 69 probands (almost all female) the frequency of nodes in th
mothers was twice that expected in the general population of comparable age, while
sisters showed a threefold increase. Stecher himself was cautious as to the form of
inheritance, but the frequent occurrence of multigeneration families led to the
assumption that autosomal dominant inheritance was acting, with the gene only
showing full penetrance by the age of 70 years in women (McKusick, 1959).

The distinction between Mendelian and polygenic inheritance in such a common
and variable trait is never simple and in particular the awkward problem of the rarit
of the condition in males has not been resolved. Some authors have postulated that
males must be homozygous to be affected (McKusick, 1959). This would imply tha
three quarters of sisters and all mothers of affected males should be affected, a read
testable situation which has apparently not been documented. An alternative sugges
tion is that hormonal or other environmental factors prevent expression of an autosomal gene in the majority of males, in which case the proportion of affected femal

186

first degree relatives of male probands would be no greater than those of female probands. In fact the limited data show the frequency in the former group to be double that in the latter (Lawrence, 1977), a finding more compatible with polygenic inheritance. Data from the same study on the incidence of generalised osteoarthrosis in relatives of probands with Heberden's nodes also fit closely with the proportion expected on the basis of polygenic inheritance.

Animal Models of Osteoarthrosis

Although inherited disorders of experimental animals may on occasion serve as useful models for comparable human disorders, they always require to be interpreted with caution. Only for genes on the X chromosome is there sufficient homology within the mammalia to be sure that a disorder studied in one species is in fact comparable to an apparently similar disorder in a different species (Ohno, 1967).

Inbred strains of the mouse have been found which show a high incidence of spontaneous osteoarthrosis and these have been extensively studied by Sokoloff and colleagues (1956, 1962). One strain (STR/IN) was characterised by severe osteoarthritis of the knees, while a second (DBA/2JN) showed a less severe form of arthritis. Sokoloff performed a number of matings which clearly showed the genetic nature of the disorder and ruled out a maternally transmitted environmental factor or sex linkage as significant factors. Unfortunately the graded nature of the arthritis, the fact that the results were expressed as mean scores for degree of arthritis rather than as individuals, and the highly inbred nature of the strain, all made it impossible to identify individual major genes which could be related to specific molecular defects. No biochemical abnormalities were found in the affected animals and although they have given a considerable amount of pathological information, their contribution to the identification of the genetic factors which are involved in human osteoarthrosis has been distinctly disappointing. A more rewarding approach could be to search for hereditary arthritis arising as new mutants in other strains of mice; the isolation of such mutants has already provided valuable information on a variety of skeletal and neurological disorders and it would be no surprise if close study of some of the already recognised skeletal mouse mutants were to reveal osteoarthrosis to be present.

A strain of 'blotchy mice' carry a gene at the 'mottled locus' of the X chromosome which manifests itself in deficient cross-linking of collagen and elastin (Rowe et al, 1974). These mice, whose enzyme defect resembles that seen in one variety of Ehlers - Danlos syndrome, develop premature osteoarthrosis of the knees (Silverberg, 1977); but it is not possible at the present time to be certain whether this is a consequence of joint hypermobility or defective bone or articular cartilage matrix.

Recent investigation of a number of strains of mice prone to auto-immune disorders has shown a high frequency of knee osteoarthrosis in NZY/B1 and PN but not NZB/B1 mice (Wigley et al, 1977). Breeding experiments suggested polygenic inheritance with at least three determining genes, and the joint disease was unrelated to any of the markers of auto-immunity.

Genetic factors are clearly important in Canine osteoarthrosis of the hip which has been widely studied in its own right rather than as a model for human disease (Lust et al, 1972; Symposium 1972; Lust and Miller, 1978). The precocious osteo-arthrosis is generally thought to be a consequence of joint subluxation and an in-born hip dysplasia with polygenic inheritance (Hutt, 1967; Leighton et al, 1977), but this remains uncertain as joint malformation is not detectable until several months after birth and as acetabular dysplasia may be a consequence rather than the cause of subluxation.

Degenerative joint disease is widespread throughout the animal kingdom, but with a few exceptions little information is available regarding the role of hereditary factors. The value of genetic analysis in domestic animals is illustrated by studies in cattle where osteoarthrosis of the stifle joints has been shown to be determined by a single recessive gene (Sittman and Kendrick, 1964) although no inborn error of metabolism has been identified to date.

Osteoarthrosis in Disorders Showing Mendelian Inheritance

Since it is clear that in the majority of cases osteoarthrosis does not follow Mendel ian inheritance, it may seem perverse to suggest that the study of Mendelian disord could shed any light on our understanding of the aetiopathogenesis of the degener-ative joint diseases as a whole. The rare inborn errors of metabolism, however, have the overwhelming advantage that they result from a single primary molecular defec of protein structure. Although such defects have only been identified in a very few cases of diseases associated with osteoarthrosis it seems highly likely that study of disorders with Mendelian inheritance offers the best chance of isolating the indiv-idual component factors that may combine to produce the commoner forms of osteoarthrosis.

Table I summarises some of the principle Mendelian disorders characterised by osteoarthrosis. Although they are a heterogeneous group of conditions in their clinical features, inheritance and the likely basis of the arthritis, several broad grou can be defined.

1. Metabolic Disorders of Connective Tissue

Alkaptonuria (Ochronosis) is the best documented example of this group. One of t original 'Inborn errors of metabolism' studied by Garrod, it provides an excellent example of how a biochemical defect in a remote organ (in this case the liver) can result in major chemical damage to essentially normal articular cartilage and other connective tissues as a secondary phenomenon. Ochronosis results from deficiency of the enzyme homogentisic acid oxidase and is transmitted by a single autosomal recessive gene (O'Brien et al, 1963). Tissue damage may result predominantly from the colourless low molecular weight oxidation product benzoquinone acetic acid which has a high binding affinity and can cross link collagen (Zannoni et al, 1962)

188

TABLE I. Some Mendelian Disorders Associated with Osteoarthrosis

Disorder	Inheritance	Reference
Heberden's Nodes	? Autosomal dominant (sex limited)	Stecher (1961)
Familial Osteoarthropathy of the fingers with avascular necrosis	Autosomal dominant	Allison and Blumberg (1958)
Interphalangeal osteo-arthrosis	Autosomal dominant	Crain (1961)
Polyarticular osteoarthrosis with platyspondyly and $\beta 2$ globulin deficiency	Autosomal recessive (probable)	Martin et al (1970)
Hereditary Arthro-ophthal-mopathy	Autosomal dominant	Stickler et al (1965)
Conradi's syndrome (chondrodysplasia punctata)	Autosomal recessive and Autosomal dominant	Tasker et al (1970)
Bone Dysplasias with short stature:		
Multiple epiphyseal dysplasia	Autosomal dominant and Autosomal recessive	Barrie et al (1958) Juberg and Holt (1965)
Pseudoachondroplasia	Autosomal dominant	Hall and Dorst (1969)
Spondyloepiphyseal dysplasia tarda	X-linked recessive	Spranger and Langer (1970)
Hereditary osteoarthrosis of the hip	Autosomal dominant	Boni (1959) Harper (1978)
Alkaptonuria	Autosomal recessive	O'Brien et al (1963)
Hereditary Chondrocalcinosis:		
Slovakian	? Autosomal recessive	Zitnan and Sitaj (1966)
Dutch	Autosomal dominant	Van der Korst et al (1974)
Chilean	Autosomal dominant	Reginato et al (1975)
Mucopolysaccharidoses		McKusick (1972)
MPS IS (Scheie	Autosomal recessive	
MPS II (Hunter)	X-linked recessive	
MPS IV (Morquio)	Autosomal recessive	

rather than from the pigmented polymers of homogentisic acid which provide the characteristic markers of the disease. It has been suggested that Alkaptonuria may be a model for other metabolic causes of osteoarthrosis which lack such an easily identifiable phenotypic marker.

The mucopolysaccharidoses (McKusick 1972) provide a further example of a group of metabolic diseases with major effects on the joints, which are of particular interest in view of the vital role of glycosaminoglycans in the structure and function of articular cartilage and synovial fluid. It is noteworthy that all the major mucopolysaccharidoses (with the exception of type IV, the Morquio Syndrome) produce a similar clinical picture of bone and joint disturbance, the clinical and radiological features being dependent more on the severity of the syndrome than on the precise biochemical defect. While more severe types such as the Hurler syndrome (MPS IH) commonly show marked changes in bony architecture, milder forms such as the Scheie syndrome (MPS IS) may show premature osteoarthrosis in the absence of structural bony abnormality. The recent identification of the specific lysosomal enzymes involved in this group of disorders, and the discovery that cells in culture express the metabolic defect, have contributed as much to our knowledge of normal connective tissue metabolism as to that of the diseases themselves.

The Morquio syndrome (MPS type IV) deserves special mention as the pattern of joint involvement is entirely different from that seen in the other mucopolysaccharidoses. Excessive joint laxity contrasts with the contractures seen in the other types, and spinal disease is prominent. Degenerative changes occur throughout the spine, but cervical spine involvement with hypoplasia of the odontoid peg, platyspondyly and altanto-axial dislocation is the major cause of death and disability. Severe osteoarthrotic changes occur in the hips and total joint replacement may be required (Jenkins et al, 1963). It seems likely that the distinctive clinical features of the Morquio syndrome are a result of an abnormality of keratan sulphate rather than dermatan sulphate metabolism; and this may well be a consequence of a chondroitin − 6 − sulphatase deficiency (Matalon et al, 1974).

Chondrocalcinosis and pseudogout are frequently associated with progressive osteoarthrosis, especially of the knees, although the wrists, metacarpophalangeal joints, hips, shoulders, elbows, ankles and spine may also be involved. Articular cartilage calcification is age related and in some patients is secondary to well defined metabolic disorders such as primary hyperparathyroidism or haemachromatosis. In the majority no specific metabolic abnormality has been defined although an abnormality of pyrophosphate metabolism is suspected (McCarty, 1976). Concentrations of inorganic pyrophosphate are increased in synovial fluid from both patients with chondrocalcinosis and simple osteoarthrosis; and pyrophosphate is released from cartilage incubates (Howell et al, 1976) but not from cell cultures of articular chondrocytes (Lust et al, 1976). Chondrocalcinosis occurs in both sporadic and familial forms. It offers an excellent example of how genetic susceptibility and a variety of environmental factors can combine to lead to premature osteoarthrosis. It also provides an excellent example of the extent of genetic heterogeneity which may underly an apparently uniform phenotypic marker. In pedigrees described in Holland (Van der Korst et al, 1974) and the Chiloe islands (Reginato et al, 1975) male to male transmission suggests autosomal dominant inheritance. This is not seen however in families from Slovakia, where homozygotes appear to have a more severe arthritis and heterozygotes a milder disease (Zitnan and Sitaj, 1966). Moreover, the disease in these families alone appears to be associated with the HL−A2, W5 haplotype (Nyulassy et al, 1976).

2. Disorders of Epiphyseal Formation

The necessity for a normally formed epiphysis if premature degeneration of weight bearing joints is to be avoided is well illustrated by the regular occurrence of arthritis in a member of inherited disorders involving epiphyseal development. This is seen most clearly in such generalised disorders as multiple epiphyseal dysplasia, where not only is there a high incidence of osteoarthrosis, but also of avascular necrosis of the hip in childhood. Among the other bone dysplasias it is those involving the epiphysis, such as pseudoachondroplasia and the various spondyloepiphyseal dysplasias that are particularly prone to severe arthritis, whereas dysplasias mainly involving the metaphyseal regions are less often characterised by this complication.

Multiple epiphyseal dysplasia (Barrie et al, 1958) is the commonest of the generalised dysplasias characterised by premature arthritis, and is also the most likely to be misdiagnosed, since stature is often only moderately reduced and may be normal. Some patients present in childhood with pain, usually in the hip, and may be misdiagnosed as Perthes disease (Figure 1). The occurrence of bilateral 'Perthes disease' with accompanying architectural abnormality of the femoral heads should raise suspicion of a more general disorder such as multiple epiphyseal dysplasia, and should prompt a skeletal survey and careful study of the family. Inheritance is characteristically autosomal dominant, but clinically indistinguishable families with recessive inheritance have been described (Juberg and Holt, 1968).

Pseudoachondroplasia is characterised by dysplasia of the spinal as well as the long bone epiphyses and is also a heterogeneous condition; with at least four distinctive types (Hall and Dorst, 1969). Pseudoachondroplastic dysplasia is frequently accompanied by severe arthritic changes in adult life. Although the limb shortening and disproportion may be partly responsible for this it is likely that other factors contribute, including the ligamentous hypermobility that characterises the disorder. Recently, Maroteaux et al (1974) have described an abnormality of proteoglycan structure in the cartilage of an affected patient, and if this can be confirmed it will be the first step in our understanding of the metabolic basis of the dominantly inherited bone dysplasias.

A third generalised dysplasia characterised by severe osteoarthrosis of hips and spine is the X-linked recessive 'tarda' form of spondyloepiphyseal dysplasia. The inheritance pattern and the characteristic radiological changes in the spine produce a specific diagnostic picture in this disorder (Figure 2) whose metabolic basis so far remains entirely unknown. A clinically distinct, autosomal recessive form of late spondyloepiphyseal dysplasia in which platyspondyly and polyarticular osteoarthrosis are associated with deficiency of β_2 Globulin, has also been described (Martin et al, 1970).

A somewhat different form of epiphyseal damage is seen in Conradi's syndrome (chondrodysplasia punctata) where widespread patchy calcification in articular and other cartilage is seen in infancy, along with shortening and asymmetry of the limbs. Although the calcification later gives way to a relatively normal appearance of ossification, premature arthritis is nonetheless a major problem in adult

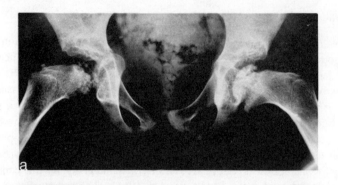

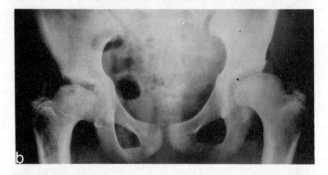

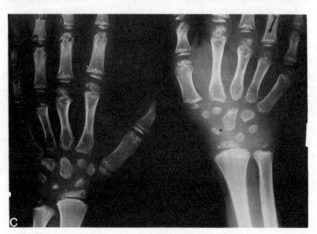

Figure 1. Multiple epiphyseal dysplasia presenting as 'Perthes Disease.'
  a) Radiograph of pelvis at time of presentation in a girl aged 10 years. There is fragment-ation of the femoral capital epiphyses and splaying of the metaphyses
  b) Radiograph of the pelvis of the same girl aged 16. There is gross flattening of the femoral heads with widening and shortening of the femoral necks and early degenerative changes
  c) Radiograph of hand of same girl aged 13 years. Multiple epiphyseal abnormalities are clearly evident

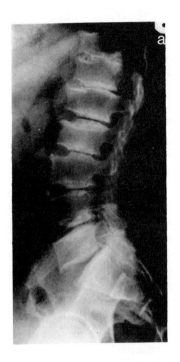

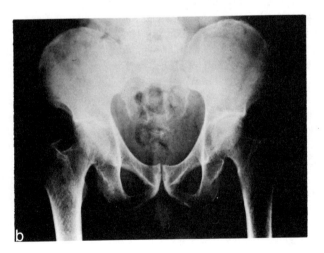

Figure 2. X-linked spondyloepiphyseal dysplasia tarda
  a) Lateral radiograph of lumbar spine of 46 year old male. The vertebrae show a characteristic hump shaped mound of dense bone in the central and posterior portions of the vertebral bodies. The disc spaces are narrowed and there are secondary degenerative changes
  b) Radiograph of the pelvis of the same patient showing narrowing, sclerosis and subchondral cyst formation in the hips associated with some splaying of the femoral heads

life. The frequent association of other general abnormalities such as mental retard-ation, cataract and ichthyosis makes a generalised metabolic defect probable in this condition, and it is of particular interest that an identical clinical picture or 'phenocopy' has been found to result from maternal warfarin therapy during preg-nancy. If the mechanism for this can be identified it may provide a valuable clue to both the pathogenesis of the genetic syndrome and the normal process of calci-fication in articular cartilage. Hereditary progressive arthro-ophthalmopathy is a further autosomal dominant disorder in which ocular abnormalities (progressive myopia) are associated with multiple epiphyseal dysplasia and premature osteo-arthrosis (Stickler et al, 1965).

Joint Hypermobility

A generalised hypermobility of joints is a feature of numerous generalised bone and connective tissue disorders, and is a common finding in normal individuals (Wynne-Davies, 1973). It is likely that it is one of the factors involved in con-genital dislocation of the hip (Carter and Wilkinson, 1964) and recurrent disloc-ations of the shoulder and patella (Carter and Sweetman, 1960). In many families the inheritance of hypermobility follows an autosomal dominant pattern (Beighton and Horan, 1970) but recessive inheritance is also encountered (Horan and Beighton, 1973). It has been suggested that hypermobility may be a major predisposing factor in osteoarthrosis (Grahame, 1978), but this view deserves a critical assess-ment before it is accepted.

About 10% of otherwise normal subjects have clinically defined evidence of joint hypermobility (Carter and Wilkinson, 1964; Beighton et al, 1973) and are prone to a variety of recurrent articular complaints which have been termed the 'hypermobility syndrome' (Kirk et al, 1967). These appear to occur in direct proportion to the degree of hypermobility (Beighton et al, 1973). However, symptoms decrease with age and decreasing mobility and they are not followed by crippling osteoarthrosis.

Table II shows some of the inherited disorders associated with joint hyper-mobility and the occurrence of arthritis in these conditions. In some, such as the generalised bone dysplasias, there are clearly other reasons for the occurrence of arthritis, and it is of note that in other dysplasias such as classical achondro-plasia, where disproportion of bone growth and hypermobility are marked, but epiphyseal development is normal, premature osteoarthrosis does not occur, though other problems such as spinal stenosis may be seen.

The inherited connective tissue disorders, including the Marfan syndrome, homocystinuria, hyperlysinaemia, pseudo-xanthoma elasticum, osteogenesis imperfecta and the Ehlers-Danlos syndrome, show joint hypermobility as an integral part of the clinical picture, and it might be expected that a high inci-dence of premature osteoarthrosis would be seen in them if hypermobility is indeed a major factor in its production. This is not the case: early osteoarthrosis is not a feature of the Marfan syndrome, homocystinuria, hyperlysinaemia,

TABLE II. Some Genetic Disorders Accompanied by Joint Hypermobility

Disorder	Inheritance	OA	Reference
Familial joint laxity	Heterogeneous	?	Wynne-Davies 1973
Homocystinuria	Autosomal recessive	-	
Marfan syndrome	Autosomal dominant	-	
Ehlers Danlos syndrome	Heterogeneous	+	Beighton 1970
Congenital dislocation of hip	Polygenic	+	
Achondroplasia	Autosomal dominant	-	
Pseudoachondroplasia	Autosomal dominant	+	
Morquio syndrome (MPS IV)	Autosomal recessive	+	McKusick 1972
Neuromuscular disorders congenital myopathies	Heterogeneous	-	
Benign spinal muscular atrophies	Autosomal recessive	-	
Downs syndrome	Chromosomal defect	-	Roberts et al 1978

pseudo-xanthoma elasticum or osteogenesis imperfecta (McKusick, 1972) while in the Ehlers-Danlos syndrome the study of Beighton (1970) showed few individuals over the age of 40 significantly disabled by osteoarthrosis, though the majority (16 out of 22) showed some radiological evidence of degenerative joint disease in at least one joint. The hips in particular were spared.

Joint hypermobility is a feature of many neuromuscular disorders of infancy, including myopathies and anterior horn cell disorders, and it may be difficult to distinguish hypotonia of neurological origin from that ensuing from a primary connective tissue defect. Although many of these disorders are either fatal or limit mobility, osteoarthrosis has not been noted in them. The same applies to the hypermobility seen in Down's syndrome, where with increasing survival osteoarthrosis might be expected to be a major problem in adult life. Although occasional instances occur, they are the exception. An observation of severe bilateral osteoarthrosis of the hip in a 30 year old female with Down's syndrome prompted a survey of the incidence of arthritis in adult patients with Down's syndrome in patients from hospitals and in the community (Roberts et al, 1978). This showed a variety of minor pelvic abnormalities, but no evidence of a major increase in generalised osteoarthrosis. Taken as a whole then, the evidence that joint hypermobility is an important factor in osteoarthrosis in man seems poor, and it is likely that it is at most a subsidiary factor.

Perthes Disease

There is no doubt that osteochondritis of the femoral capital epiphysis in childhood can lead to osteoarthrosis of the hip in later life. It seems likely however that the genetic component of Perthes disease has been considerably overestimated, possibly by the inclusion of such Mendelian disorders as multiple epiphyseal dysplasia. Although early surveys (Wansbrough et al, 1959) suggested a considerably increased incidence among relatives, recent more detailed genetic studies have shown the risk to be only slightly increased, even for first degree relatives (Gray et al, 1972; Harper et al, 1976). Frequent discordance in monozgotic twin pairs also suggests a relatively minor hereditary component and new data on the offspring of affected individuals which is now becoming available tends to confirm this (Table III).

TABLE III. Genetic Risks in Perthes' Disease

All cases	Total number of probands 120		
	Total	*affected*	*% affected*
Sibs	323	2	0.62
Children	77(35.3)*	1	1.30 (2.83)*
Parents	240	0	0
2nd degree relatives	1171	2	0.18

Unilateral	Total number of probands 104		
	Total	*affected*	*% affected*
Sibs	269	2	0.74
Children	74(35.3)*	1	1.35 (2.83)*
Parents	208	0	0
2nd degree relatives	989	1	0.10

Bilateral	Total number of probands 16		
	Total	*affected*	*% affected*
Sibs	54	0	0
Children	3(0)*	0	0
Parents	32	0	0
2nd degree relatives	182	1	0.55

*Figures in parenthesis are adjusted for age on onset. From Harper et al (1976)

Osteochondritis and Avascular Necrosis

Avascular necrosis is considered to be the principal aetiological factor in Perthes disease of childhood as the lesion can be reproduced in experimental animals by occlusion of the blood supply to the femoral capital epiphysis. Osteochondritis affecting a number of other epiphyses is usually assumed to have a similar pathogenesis: e.g. Osgood - Schlatter's disease affecting the epiphysis of the tibial tubercle, Kohler's disease affecting the tarsal navicular, Scheuermann's disease affecting the vertebral bodies, Panner's disease affecting the elbow, Kienbock's disease affecting the lunate and Haglund's disease affecting the calcaneum. However, genetic factors and trauma have also been implicated in the pathogenesis of these lesions and in *osteochondritis dissecans*. The latter condition in particular, which is characterised by separation of a piece of articular cartilage and underlying bone most commonly from the medial femoral condyle or the capitellum of the humerus, has been noted to occur in multiple generations of the same family (Stougaard, 1964). If left untreated, it frequently leads to osteoarthrosis.

Avascular necrosis of the epiphyses at the interphalangeal joints of the fingers (Desseker, 1930) and the metatarsophalangeal joints of the toes is probably the underlying cause of *Thiemann's disease,* a rare familial condition with autosomal dominant inheritance that may be mistaken for primary generalised osteoarthrosis (Rubinstein, 1975). Other families have been reported where osteoarthrosis is mainly confined to the fingers.

Two families reported by Allison and Blumberg (1958) showed clear autosomal dominant inheritance. In one, the child of a marriage between affected subjects was severely affected suggesting homozygosity.

The pathology in other families with a superficially similar condition (Crain, 1961) may well be different. Largely because of the radiological appearances such patients are often described as having 'erosive osteoarthritis' (Peter et al, 1966), and clinical and histological studies in similar but non-familial sporadic cases suggest a recurrent low grade synovitis.

Hereditary Osteoarthrosis of the Hips

Analysis of X-rays of 200 adults presenting to an orthopaedic hospital in London with 'primary' osteoarthrosis suggested that in 25% the disease was a consequence of acetabular dysplasia, and that in 40% it was associated with a 'tilt deformity' as a consequence of minor epiphysiolysis (Murray, 1965). Genetic factors are certainly important determinants of acetabular dysplasia whose incidence varies considerably in different ethnic groups. Figures as high as 57% and 48% have been reported from Northern Italy (Calandriello, 1963) and Norway (Gade, 1947) respectively while primary coxarthrosis and hip dysplasia are almost unheard of in the African Bantu (Solomon et al, 1975; Roper, 1976).

Although osteoarthrosis of the hips is a feature of a number of genetic syndromes, and may be the presenting complaint in some of these, the existence of a specific Mendelian disorder in which significant abnormalities are confined to the hips does not seem to be generally recognised. A number of early reports exist of 'familial' osteoarthrosis of the hip and familial Perthes disease which probably represent multiple epiphyseal dysplasia (Stephens and Kerby, 1946; Monty, 1962), but that a separate disorder not affecting stature and without clinical evidence of generalised epiphyseal involvement exists is shown by the unusual family described below.

The propositus of the family, a university lecturer, aged 28, was originally seen for genetic counselling for 'Perthes disease.' Closer enquiry showed that both he and his brother had been treated in childhood for this disorder by prolonged traction; symptoms in the propositus had begun aged 7 years, with pain in the left hip, and at this age both femoral heads showed radiological evidence of fragmentation and flattening. Surgery for removal of a loose body from the left hip had been required aged 10 years, but he had remained well subsequently, with pain in the hips only after excessive exercise, and no symptoms referrable to other joints. When examined aged 28 years he showed marked reduction in movements at both hips but no evidence of involvement of other joints or of the spine. Stature was normal and there were no abnormalities of other systems. Enquiry into the family produced the remarkable pedigree of hip disease shown in Figure 3. Apart from

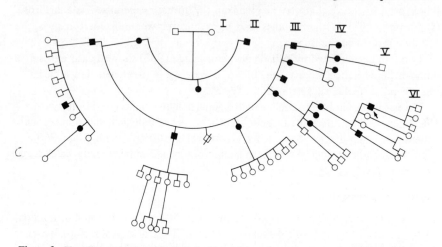

Figure 3. Hereditary osteoarthritis of the hips. An autosomal dominant pattern of inheritance is seen in this family whose members presented with bilateral hip disease in the absence of clinical involvement of other joints

the brother of the propositus, affected individuals had not presented in childhood as 'Perthes disease', but as premature bilateral osteoarthrosis of the hip, requiring hip replacement in at least three instances. Radiographic appearances of the hips in affected members are shown in Figures 4a and 4b. No individuals had clinical evidence of involvement of other joints, and none had unusually short stature, while lifespan appeared unaffected.

The mode of inheritance in this family is clearly autosomal dominant, though some branches have yet to be fully documented. There seems equally little doubt that the disorder is not true Perthes disease, nor is it multiple epiphyseal dysplasia, but a distinct Mendelian disorder with clinical manifestations confined to the hips. A similar family has been described by Boni (1959).

No metabolic basis has yet been found (mucopolysaccharide excretion in the propositus was normal) and it remains uncertain whether the primary defect lies in the morphology of the femoral head or acetabulum, or whether it results from

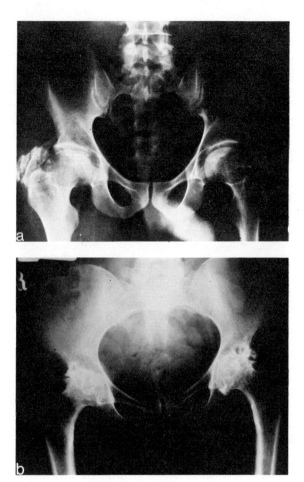

Figure 4.
    a) Hereditary osteoarthritis of the hips. Radiograph of hips of propositus aged 28. Both
hips show dysplastic and degenerative changes. Right hip shows abnormal bone formation
following surgery and immobilisation in childhood for removal of loose body
    b) Radiograph of pelvis of maternal aunt of propositus prior to bilateral hip replacement

a defective blood supply leading to avascular necrosis. As an example of a 'pure'
type of osteoarthrosis this disorder provides a potentially valuable model in investigating the factor underlying osteoarthrosis in general.

Conclusions

The genetic basis for osteoarthrosis in man remains poorly understood. Family
and epidemiological studies of the disorder in the general population have indicated
that important genetic influences do exist, but that osteoarthrosis in general does

not follow patterns of simple Mendelian inheritance. Apart from the relationship with Heberden's nodes, where Mendelian inheritance is possible though not proven, no individual genes have been identified which can be stated with certainty to be acting in the production of osteoarthrosis, nor has comparable information so far come from the use of experimental animal models. By contrast, a number of genetic disorders showing clear Mendelian inheritance are recognised in which arthritis is a major feature, and in some of these the underlying changes responsible for the joint disease are at least partially understood. Analysis of these disorders shows a variety of mechanisms to be responsible for osteoarthrosis occurring in them. While there is no direct evidence that these actual genes are operating in the causation of osteoarthrosis in general, the fact that a single primary abnormality is likely to be operating in each Mendelian disorder makes identification of important causative factors a feasible objective. As our knowledge of these individual components increases, we may be able to assess more clearly their relative importance in osteoarthrosis as a whole, where both the genetic and environmental factors are complex and elusive.

References

Allison, AC and Blumberg, FS (1958) *Journal of Bone and Joint Surgery, 40B*, 538
Barrie H, Carter, C and Sutcliffe, J (1958) *British Medical Journal, 2*, 133
Beighton, P (1970) *The Ehlers-Danlos Syndrome*, Heinemann, London
Beighton, P and Horan, F (1970) *Journal of Bone and Joint Surgery, 52B*, 145
Beighton, P, Solomon, L and Soskolne, CL (1973) *Annals of the Rheumatic Diseases, 32*, 413
Boni, A (1959) *Seminar International, 8*, 16
Calandriello, B (1963) *The Epidemiology of Chronic Rheumatism, Vol. I*, Pages 122-127
    Blackwell, Oxford
Canine Hip Dysplasia Symposium and Workshop (1972) *Orthopaedic Foundation for Animals*
Carter, CO (1969) *British Medical Bulletin, 25*, 52
Carter, CS and Sweetman, R (1960) *Journal of Bone and Joint Surgery, 42B*, 183
Carter, CS and Wilkinson, J (1964) *Journal of Bone and Joint Surgery, 46B*, 40
Crain, DC (1967) *Journal of American Medical Association, 175*, 1049
Desseker, C (1930) *Deutsche Zeitschrift fur chirugie, 229*, 327
Ercilla, MG, Brancos, MA, Breysse, Y, Alonso, G, Vives, J, Castillo, R and Querol, JR (1977)
    Journal of Rheumatology, 4, 89
Falconer, DS (1965) *Annals of Human Genetics, 29*, 51
Gade, HG (1947) *Acta Chirurgica Scandinavica, 95, Suppl. 120*, 32
Grahame, R (1978) In *Copemans Textbook of Rheumatic Diseases.* (Ed) JT Scott, 5th Ed.,
    Churchill Livingstone, London, Page 835
Gray, IM, Lowry, RB and Renwick, DHG (1972) *Journal of Medical Genetics, 9*, 197
Hall, JG and Dorst, JP (1969) In *Clinical Delineation of Birth Defects Part IV Dysplasias.*
    (Ed) D Bergsma - National Foundation - March of Dimes. New York, Page 242
Harper, PS, Brotherton, BJ and Cochlin, D (1976) *Clinical Genetics, 10*, 178
Hermann, R (1936) *Zeitschrifte fur Menschliche Kunstlehre, 19*, 707
Horan, F and Beighton, P (1973) *Rheumatology and Rehabilitation, 12*, 47
Howell, DS, Muniz, O, Pita, JC and Enis, JE (1976) *Arthritis and Rheumatism, 19*, 488
Hutt, FB (1967) *Journal of the American Veterinary Association, 151*, 1041
Jenkins, P, Davies, GR and Harper, PS (1973) *British Journal of Radiology, 46*, 668
Juberg, RC and Holt, JF (1968) *American Journal of Human Genetics, 20*, 549
Kellgren, JH, Lawrence, JS and Bier, F (1963) *Annals of the Rheumatic Diseases, 22*, 237
Kellgren, JH and Moore, R (1952) *British Medical Journal, 1*, 181

King, JB (1968) *Arthritis and Rheumatism Council Annual Report,* Page 66

Kirk, JA, Ansell, BM and Bywaters, EGTL (1967) *Annals of the Rheumatic Diseases, 26,* 419

Lawrence, JS (1977) *Rheumatism in Populations.* Heinemann, London

Leighton, EA, Linn, JM, Willham, RL and Castleberry, MW (1977) *American Journal of Veterinary Research, 38,* 241

Lust, G and Miller, DR (1979) In *Models for Osteoarthrosis.* (Ed) G Nuki. Pitman Medical Tunbridge Wells (In press)

Lust, G, Nuki, G and Seegmiller, JE (1976) *Arthritis and Rheumatism, 19,* 479

Lust, G, Pronsky, W and Sherman, DM (1972) *American Journal of Veterinary Research, 33,* 2429

McCarty, DJ (1976) *Arthritis and Rheumatism, 19,* 275

McKusick, V (1959) *American Journal of Medicine, 26,* 283

McKusick, VA (1972) *Hereditable Disorders of Connective Tissue,* 4th Ed. St Louis. Mosby

Stanescu, V and Maroteaux, P (1973) *Comptes Rendues: Acadamie de Sciences, 277,* 2585

Martin, JR, Macewan, DW, Blais, JA, Metrakos, J, Gold, P, Langer, F and Hill, RO (1970) *Arthritis and Rheumatism, 13,* 53

Matalon, R, Arbogast, B, Justice, P and Dorfman, A (1974) *Biochemical Biophysical Research Communications, 61,* 1450

Murray, RO (1965) *British Journal of Radiology, 38,* 810

Nyulassy, S, Stefanovic, J, Sitaj, S and Zitnan, D (1976) *Arthritis and Rheumatism, 19,* 391

O'Brien, WM, La Du, BN and Bunim, JJ (1963) *American Journal of Medicine, 34,* 813

Ohno, S (1967) *Sex-chromosomes and Sex-linked Genes,* Springer, Berlin

Peter, JB, Pearson, CM and Marmor, L (1966) *Arthritis and Rheumatism, 9,* 365

Reginato, AJ, Hollander, JL and Martinez, V (1975) *Annals of the Rheumatic Diseases, 34,* 260

Roper, A (1976) *Journal of Bone and Joint Surgery, 58B,* 155

Rowe, DW, McGoodwin, EB, Martin, GR, Sussman, MD, Grahn, D, Faris, B and Franzblan, C, *Journal of Experimental Medicine, 139,* 180

Rubenstein, HM (1975) *Arthritis and Rheumatism, 18,* 357

Silberberg, R (1977) *Experimental Cell Biology, 45,* 1

Sittman, K and Kendrick, JW (1964) *Genetica, 35,* 132

Sokoloff, L (1956) *American Medical Association Archives of Pathology, 62,* 118

Sokoloff, L, Crittenden, LB, Yamamoto, RS and Jay, GE Jnr. (1962) *Arthritis and Rheumatism, 5,* 531

Solomon, L, Beighton, P and Lawrence, JS (1975) *South African Medical Journal, 49,* 1737

Spranger, JW and Langer, LO (1970) *Radiology, 94,* 313

Stecher, RM (1941) *American Journal of Medical Sciences, 201,* 801

Stecher, RM (1955) *Annals of the Rheumatic Diseases, 14,* 1

Stickler, GB, Belan, PG, Farrell, FJ, Jones, JD, Pugh, DG, Steinberg, AG and Ward, LE (1965) *Mayo Clinic Proceedings, 40,* 433

Stoia, I, Ramneautu, R and Poitas, M (1967) *Annals of the Rheumatic Diseases, 26,* 332

Stougaard, J (1964) *Journal of Bone and Joint Surgery, 46B,* 542

Tasker, WG, Mastri, AR and Gold, AP (1970) *American Journal of Diseases of Children, 119,* 122

Van der Korst, JA, Geerards, J and Driessens, FCM (1974) *American Journal of Medicine, 56,* 307

Wansborough, RM, Carrie, AW, Walker, NF and Ruckerbauer, G (1959) *Journal of Bone and Joint Surgery, 41A,* 135

Wigley, RD, Couchman, JG, Maule, R and Reay, BR (1977) *Annals of the Rheumatic Diseases, 36,* 249

Wynne-Davies, R (1973) *Hereditable Disorders in Orthopaedic Practice,* Blackwell Scientific Publications, Oxford

Zannoni, VG, Malawista, SE and La Du, BN (1962) *Arthritis and Rheumatism, 5,* 547

Zitnan, D and Sitaj, S (1966) *Acta Rheumatologica et Balneologica Pistiniana, 2,* 9

SUBJECT INDEX

abbreviations   OA   Osteoarthrosis/Osteoarthritis
                       GAG   Glycosaminoglycan

Abrader, abrasive damage
  see Mechanical injury
Acetic acid, benzoquinone, and tissue
  damage in ochronosis, 188
Accidents and OA, 85
Acetabular dysplasia and OA, 197
Achondroplasia and OA, 194
Acid phosphatase
  see Phosphatase, acid
Acromegaly
  and cartilage stress, 86
  and OA, 66
  as cause of OA, 93
Actinomycin D and pyrophosphate, 99
Age of onset secondary and idiopathic OA
  compared, 148, 149, 152
Ageing
  biological, 9
  and cartilage senescence, 12
  cartilage and, 75, 76–78, 82
  cellular senescence, 9–10
  changes
    as cause of OA, 1–14, 85, 94, 95,
    125
    distinction from OA, 7
    OA
      role in, 1–14
      semantic problems, 8–9
  pathological, 9, 13
Albumin, serum and OA cartilage, 43
Alkaline phosphatase
  see Phosphatase, alkaline
Alkaptonuria
  see Ochronosis
American Indians, OA patterns, 178, 180,
  181, 182
Amianthoid degeneration, 11
Amino acids, and proteoglycan synthesis,
  126
Amino sugars
  content in cartilage in exp. canine OA, 55,
    59, 60
  and proteoglycan synthesis, 126

Amyloid deposits in OA, 8
Anatomical abnormalities
  see Dysplasia
Apatite
  see also Hydroxyapatite
  and chondrocalcinosis, 97, 98, 102
  crystal deposition, 114, 115
  formation in matrix vesicles, 107
Arteries, occlusion in OA, 4
Arthro-ophthalmopathy, hereditary, and
  OA, 189, 194
Articular cartilage
  see Cartilage, articular
Aryl sulphatase activity in extracellular
  vesicles in cartilage, 106
Asbestoid degeneration, 11
Aseptic necrosis, in OA, 4
ATPase in matrix vesicles in cartilage, 107
Autoantibody reactivity in secondary and
  idiopathic OA, 149, 152, 153
Avascular necrosis
  in familial osteoarthropathy of fingers
    and OA, 189
  and OA, 196–197
  and pyrophosphate, 99

Baker's cysts in OA, 119
Benzoquinone acetic acid and tissue damage
  in ochronosis, 188
Biochemical
  aetiological factors in OA, 93
  changes in canine OA, 47–51
  induction in OA, 125
  manipulation and cure for OA, 35
  studies of OA cartilage, 37–45
Biochemistry, macromolecular,of cartilage,
  52–64
Blood groups and OA, 186
Body build and OA, 179
Bone
  see also Subchondral bone

203

Bone *(continued)*
  deformation and cartilage stress, 86
  in late-stage OA, histological pattern, 18
  necrosis in OA, 4–5
  subchondral
    see Subchondral bone
Bouchard's nodes, 118
Bumadizone to induce exp. OA, 127
Buttress osteophyte, 3, 7

Calcification
  of cartilage, 95–96, 99–100
    epiphyseal, 106–107
  disorders as cause of OA, 94
  mechanisms
    in cartilage, OA, 113–114
    in cell culture, alteration, 100
Calcium
  chloride and proteoglycans, 57
  concentration by matrix vesicles, 107
  phosphate and OA, 96, 97
  storage in cartilage, 101
Callus reaction in subchondral marrow, 4
Car accidents and OA, 85
Cartilage
  age, variations, 75, 76–78
  breakdown
    bone exposure prior to, in late stage,
      OA, 18
    causes, 44
    cycle of, 25
    intermediate stage OA, 20–23
    in OA, 16–28
  calcification
    see Calcification of cartilage
  chemical composition in OA, 37
  compliance in articular, 75–78
  composition, articular, 79–81
  degeneration
    in articular, 1–4
    exp. OA, 136–137
  density of OA, 40, 42, 66
  destructive element in OA, 16–28
  detachment in articular, 4
  elastic properties, 2
    and calcium, 114
    in articular and OA, 65
  epiphyseal,calcification, 106–107
  in exp. canine OA, 55–57
  fibre network, fatigue strength, and
    cartilage breakdown, 90
  fibrillation
    see Fibrillation
  hollows in surface, 69, 71, 72

Cartilage *(continued)*
  human femoral head, studies on articular,
    65–81
  macromolecular biochemistry, 52–64
  mass in normal hip joints, 66
  matrix vesicles
    function in articular, 107–113
    mineral-containing in human,
      105–115
    pictures, 108–112
    structure, 108–112
  mechanical failure of articular, causes of,
    79
  metabolism, biochemical changes, drug-
    induced, 123–138
  mineralisation and OA, 93–102
  in normal hip joints, 66
  osteoarthrotic,
    biochemical studies, 37–45
    density, 40, 42
    destructive element in, 16–28
    pathophysiology, 124
    physico-chemical studies, 37–45
    physico-chemical properties and
      chemical composition, 41
  physiology, 123–124
  pigmentation of senescent, 12
  removal, complete, and cartilage wear, 87
  scarification, experimental, 17, 23
  senescence and biological ageing, 12
  as shock absorber, articular, 5
  splitting of uncalcified, 19, 20, 21
  stress
    see Stress
  superficial tangential layer, role in OA, 4
  surface of articular
    grading in experimental OA, 54
    structure, 67–69
  swelling characteristics, 39, 43, 91, 114,
    119, 121
  tensile strength, loss of, 90
  thickness
    of articular, 69–75
    before fibrillation, 91
    and cartilage damage, 26
    in normal hip joints, 66
  ultrastructure, articular, 105–106
  wear, causes, 86–88
    as precursor of OA, 24
Cathepsin
  B and collagen in cartilage in OA, 91
  D in animal cartilage, and cause of OA,
    95
Cathepsins
  in OA, 10
Caucasian populations and OA, 180–181

204

205

Debris, lipidic, in cartilage, 106
Dermatosporaxis and procollagen, 51
Developmental
  causes of OA, 84
  errors as cause of OA, 94
Dexamethasone-O-phosphate to induce exp.
  OA, 127
Dicalcium phosphate dihydrate in cartilage,
  114
Diet and OA, 179
DNA content of OA cartilage, 48, 133–134
Dog, suitability for experimental OA, 52
Down's Syndrome and OA, 195
Drug-induced
  biochemical changes in cartilage metab-
    olism, 123–138
  cartilage inhibition, 125–127
Drugs, anti-inflammatory and anti-rheumatic,
  connective tissue metabolism and
  induction of OA, 126
Dysplasia
  acetabular, and OA, 197
  bone with short stature and OA, 189, 191
  chondro-
    see Conradi's syndrome
  complex deposition in OA secondary to,
    147
  multiple epiphysial, 47
  as precursor of OA, 24, 124
  pseudoachondroplastic, proteoglycan
    structure in, 191
  and stress on cartilage, 85

Eburnation in advanced OA, 2, 3, 4
Effusion in OA, 8, 119
Ehlers-Danlos syndrome
  as cause of OA, 93
  mouse enzyme defect resembling, 187
  and OA, 194, 195
  type VII and procollagen, 51
Elastin and collagen, deficient cross-linking
  in OA, 187
Endocrine
  abnormalities and cartilage stress, 86
  diseases and OA, 66, 94
English populations and OA patterns, 178,
  180, 181, 182
Environmental factors and OA, 184, 185
Enzymatic
  disorders as cause of OA, 94
  origin of OA, 66
Enzyme activity in articular cartilage, 113
Enzymes
  and cartilage breakdown, 84
  degradative in OA, 31

Epiphyseal
  cartilage calcification, 106–107
  dysplasia, multiple, 47
  formation,disorders of, 191–194
ESR
  see Sedimentation rate

Factory workers and OA, 180
Familial disease
  see Genetic disease
'Fatigue failure' of collagen fibre framework,
  26
Fatigue in sequence of OA, 11
Femoral head, osteoarthrotic cartilage,
  studies, 37
Fibrillation
  and cartilage
    breakdown, 84, 90–91
    in intermediate stage OA, 20
    wear, 86
  and chemical composition of cartilage,
    39, 40, 41
  development with age, 2
  and fatigue failure of collagen fibre
    framework, 26
  in OA, and collagen, 11
  as starting point of OA, 12
Fibrosis in advanced OA, 8
Fishermen and OA, 180
Flufenamic acid to induce exp. OA, 127, 129
Fluoride and OA, 181
Footwear and OA, 181
Fracture
  of bone and cartilage stress, 86
  femoral neck, 99
Fractures, minute, in subchondral bone,
  4, 65
Free radicals and cause of OA, 94, 95

GAG
  see Glycosaminoglycan
Galactosamine, content of cartilage in exp.
  canine OA, 55, 59, 60
Galactose, content of cartilage in exp.
  canine OA, 33, 55
Galenic signs of inflammation, 121
Ganglia and subchondral pseudocysts, 7
Gaucher's disease and cartilage stress, 86
Genes, individual, in generalised OA, 186
Genetic
  causes
    of OA, 65, 84, 93, 179, 184–200
    in OA, animal models, 187

206

208

Necrosis
see Aseptic necrosis; Avascular necrosis;
Bone necrosis; Cell necrosis
Negroes, OA patterns, 179, 180, 181, 182
Neurogenic disease, complex deposition in
OA secondary to, 147
Neuromuscular disorders of infancy and OA,
195
Neuronal diseases and OA, 66
Niflumic acid to induce exp. OA, 127, 135
Nucleotides
cyclic in chondrocyte metabolism 95
metabolism in cartilage, 100–101
Nucleus, anti-nuclear factor and idiopathic
OA, 148–149
Nutritional requirements of articular cartilage
and OA, 124, 125, 137

Obesity and OA, 125
Occupational factors in OA, 162, 167, 179,
180
Ochronosis
and cartilage stress, 86
as cause of OA, 93
and OA, 24
OA in, 188–189
Ollier's disease as cause of OA, 93
Ophthalmopathy, arthro-, hereditary, and OA,
189, 194
Osgood-Schatter's disease, 196
Osmotic pressure in OA cartilage, 42, 43–44
Osteoarthritis
see Osteoarthrosis
Osteoarthropathy, familial of fingers, and
OA, 189
Osteoarthrosis
advanced, appearance, 2, 3
aetiology, 50, 65–66
calcification mechanisms and, 113–114
biochemical changes, 29–35
canine, natural and experimental, 55
carpo-metacarpal joints, geography,
169–171, 180, 181
cure for, hypothesis, 35
definition, 8–9
demographic features, 148, 152, 155–182
of distal interphalangeal joints, geography,
162–164, 180
duration of disease, idiopathic and
secondary compared, 149, 152
'erosive', 118
experimental, biochemical changes,
timing, 63–64
experimental, canine, 47–51, 52–64
as final common pathway, 84–88

Osteoarthrosis *(continued)*
genetic factors, 100, 184–200
geography, 155–182
heterogeneity, 23–24
of the hip
canine genetic factors in, 188
geography, 172–174, 182
hereditary, 197–199
idiopathic
immunoglobulins and complement
components in, 144–153
pathogenesis, 90–92
inflammatory, 153
component, 117–122
interphalangeal, 189
inflammation in, 118
of knees, geography, 174–175, 182
laboratory and demographic features
compared, 148, 152
late-stage cartilage destruction in, 17–19
mechanisms involved, 1
metacarpophalangeal joints, geography,
166–168, 180
metatarsophalangeal joints, first,
geography, 175–179, 181, 182
multiple aetiological factors, 93–94
nodal, and non-nodal generalised,
geography, 161, 180, 181, 182
pathology, 1–14
polyarticular, 117–118
with platyspondyly and B2 globulin
deficiency, 189, 191
pre-clinical, 23–28
precocious, genetic factors, 188
predisposing factors, 23–24, 125
primary,
see Idiopathic
progressive, non-progressive ageing
changes in cartilage, 9, 12
of proximal interphalangeal joints,
geography, 164–166
repair, 13
staging, 144–145
of wrists, geography, 171–172
Osteochondritis and OA, 196–197
Osteocytes, necrobiosis, 4–5
Osteogenesis imperfecta and OA, 194, 195
Osteopenia and cartilage stress, 86
Osteophyte
formation and OA, 162
structure in OA, 7–8
Osteophytes in advanced OA, 2,3
Osteoporosis
and cartilage stress, 86
and OA, 65
in subchondral bone in OA, 5
Osteotomy, as cure for OA, 35
Oxyphenbutazone to induce exp. OA, 127

209

Paget's disease
and cartilage stress, 86
as cause of OA, 93
Pain
in OA, 8
sensitivity and OA, 181
Panner's disease, 197
Papain, injection in rabbits to produce
experimental OA, 17
D-penicillamine to induce exp. OA, 127
Peptide, connective tissue activating
see Connective tissue activating peptide
Perthes disease
bilateral, and OA, 191, 192
and OA, 195–196, 197
Phenylbutazone to induce exp. OA, 127, 128,
130, 131, 133, 134
Phosphatase
acid
activity in extracellular vesicles in
cartilage, 106
activity in OA, 31, 32
and calcification as cause of OA, 95
in matrix vesicles in cartilage, 106
alkaline
in matrix vesicles in cartilage, 106,
113, 114, 115
in OA cartilage, 102
Phosphate, calcium and OA, 96, 97
Physico-chemical studies of OA cartilage,
37–45
Pigmentation of senescent cartilage, 12
Pituitary growth factors and cause of OA,
95
Polished appearance
see Eburnation
Polyarthritis, sero-negative, geography, 180
Polygenic inheritance in OA, 186, 187
Prenatal errors as cause of OA, 94
Pressure distribution and cartilage wear, 87
Procollagen and aetiology of OA, 50–51
^{14}C-proline
see also Collagen
incorporation into articular cartilage, 48
Prostaglandin A$_1$ and OA, 66
Prostaglandins in chondrocyte metabolism,
95
Proteases and articular chondrocytes, 10
Protein
content of cartilage in exp. canine OA,
55, 60
synthesis,
errors in, as cause of OA, 94, 95
inhibition by anti-inflammatory drugs,
126
Proteoglycan
and cartilage compliance, 78

Proteoglycan *(continued)*
content of cartilage
and age, 65
in OA, 47, 48, 133, 134
depletion in matrix in OA, 29–31
in ground substance in intermediate
stage OA, 22
ground substance in OA, 11
structure in pseudoachondroplastic
dysplasia, 191
synthesis
errors in, as cause of OA, 94, 95
inhibition by anti-inflammatory
drugs, 126, 129, 130
qualitative change in, 91
and synovial medium, 140, 141, 143
Proteoglycans
articular cartilage, composition, 80
in cartilage in exp. canine OA, 57, 58
depletion, in sequence of OA, 11
and mechanical properties of cartilage,
25
molecular size, 60
and nucleation, 101
radiosulphate in, 9
and water content of cartilage, 38, 43
Pseudoachondroplasia and OA, 191
Pseudocysts
in advanced OA, 2, 3
subchondral (geodes), 5–7
Pseudogout, 114
and chondrocalcinosis, 96
and OA, 190
Pseudo-xanthoma elasticum and OA, 194,
195
Pyrophosphatase in matrix vesicles in cartilage,
106, 115
Pyrophosphate
arthropathy and OA, 24
and cartilage mineralisation, 97–99,
100–101
crystals in OA, 119, 120, 121
metabolism and cartilage calcification,
190

Racial variations and OA, 159, 162, 169,
171, 180, 181, 182
Radiosulphate
see Sulphate
Remodelling
of bone in OA, 5, 101–102, 114
of cartilage in OA, 17
Repair
of osteoarthrosis, 11, 13
process
in cartilage in OA, 17